Psychoanalytic Psychotherapy with Adolescents

In this book, Philip Rosenbaum and Richard Webb consider the complexities of working as counselors and psychotherapists for college students, and offer a broad and detailed account of the developmental issues essential to understanding adolescent experience.

Drawing on existentialism, cultural psychology and relational and object relations theories in psychoanalysis, this book offers a perspective that is sensitive to both clinical concerns and the broader context of college counseling and working with adolescents. Particular attention is paid to the emergence of adolescent identities through a relationship with "otherness," and several considerations are explored as a result. These include the emergence and reconciliation of destructive feelings, suicidal phenomenology and the effects of trauma.

By taking a fresh look at clinical developmental theories as they affect adolescents and young adults, Rosenbaum and Webb provide a view of college-student development that is theoretically rich and clinically applicable in a way that warrants renewed appreciation and practice among counselors, psychotherapists and psychoanalysts working with college-age clients.

Philip J. Rosenbaum is a clinical psychologist, supervising psychoanalyst and the Director of Counseling and Psychological Services at Haverford College. He is the editor of the book *Making Our Ideas Clear: Pragmatism and Psychoanlaysis*, and an emeriti editor of the *Journal of College Student Psychotherapy*. He is in private practice in Philadelphia. His website is www.philiprosenbaumphd.com.

Richard E. Webb is a clinical psychologist in a private practice in Lansdale, PA (USA). He was the Director of Counseling and Psychological Services at Haverford College for 32 years. He has published in a variety of journals including the *Journal of Constructivist Psychology*, *International Journal of Psychoanalysis*, *Theory & Psychology* and *Journal of Infant, Child, and Adolescent Psychotherapy*.

Psychoanalysis in a New Key Book Series

Series Editor
Donnel Stern

When music is played in a new key, the melody does not change, but the notes that make up the composition do: change in the context of continuity, continuity that perseveres through change. Psychoanalysis in a New Key publishes books that share the aims psychoanalysts have always had, but that approach them differently. The books in the series are not expected to advance any particular theoretical agenda, although to this date most have been written by analysts from the interpersonal and relational orientations.

The most important contribution of a psychoanalytic book is the communication of something that nudges the reader's grasp of clinical theory and practice in an unexpected direction. Psychoanalysis in a New Key creates a deliberate focus on innovative and unsettling clinical thinking. Because that kind of thinking is encouraged by exploration of the sometimes surprising contributions to psychoanalysis of ideas and findings from other fields, Psychoanalysis in a New Key particularly encourages interdisciplinary studies. Books in the series have married psychoanalysis with dissociation, trauma theory, sociology and criminology. The series is open to the consideration of studies examining the relationship between psychoanalysis and any other field – for instance, biology, literary and art criticism, philosophy, systems theory, anthropology and political theory.

But innovation also takes place within the boundaries of psychoanalysis, and Psychoanalysis in a New Key therefore also presents work that reformulates thought and practice without leaving the precincts of the field. Books in the series focus, for example, on the significance of personal values in psychoanalytic practice, on the complex interrelationship between the analyst's clinical work and personal life, on the consequences for the clinical situation when patient and analyst are from different cultures, and on the need for psychoanalysts to accept the degree to which they knowingly satisfy their own wishes during treatment hours, often to the patient's detriment.

A full list of all titles in this series is available at: https://www.routledge.com/Psychoanalysis-in-a-New-Key-Book-Series/book-series/LEAPNKBS

Psychoanalytic Psychotherapy with Adolescents

College student development and treatment

Philip J. Rosenbaum and
Richard E. Webb

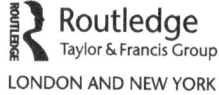
Routledge
Taylor & Francis Group

LONDON AND NEW YORK

Cover image: Photo taken by Richard Webb

First published 2022
by Routledge
4 Park Square, Milton Park, Abingdon, Oxon OX14 4RN

and by Routledge
605 Third Avenue, New York, NY 10158

Routledge is an imprint of the Taylor & Francis Group, an informa business

British Library Cataloguing-in-Publication Data
A catalogue record for this book is available from the British Library

Library of Congress Cataloguing-in-Publication Data
Names: Rosenbaum, Philip (Philip J.), 1981- author. |
Webb, Richard (Richard E.), 1951- author.
Title: Psychoanalytic psychotherapy with adolescents : college student development and treatment / Philip J. Rosenbaum, Ph.D & Richard E. Webb, Ph.D. |
Identifiers: LCCN 2021053014 (print) | LCCN 2021053015 (ebook) | ISBN 9781032159782 (hardback) |
ISBN 9781032159744 (paperback) | ISBN 9781003246558 (ebook)
Subjects: LCSH: Adolescent psychotherapy. | Adolescent psychology. | College student development programs.
Classification: LCC RJ503 .R67 2022 (print) |
LCC RJ503 (ebook) | DDC 616.89/140835--dc23/eng/20211206
LC record available at https://lccn.loc.gov/2021053014
LC ebook record available at https://lccn.loc.gov/2021053015

ISBN: 978-1-032-15978-2 (hbk)
ISBN: 978-1-032-15974-4 (pbk)
ISBN: 978-1-003-24655-8 (ebk)

DOI: 10.4324/9781003246558

Typeset in Times New Roman
by MPS Limited, Dehradun

'This is, ultimately, a book about important details of human experience. Through its exploration of work with college students in a college psychological service setting, this book succeeds at its ambitious task of illuminating all human developmental experience with both clarity and profundity. Weaving together a well-chosen and soundly integrated range of psychoanalytic, psychodynamic, existential-humanistic, and pragmatic approaches, with an accessible Interpersonal-Relational sensibility, this book contributes cutting edge thought and practical guidance on working with this always-compelling, often fraught, adolescent-through-young-adult, college student population.

The authors' experience and wisdom in working with college students while resourcefully engaging with the structures and systems within which this work occurs shines throughout this readable and reflection-inspiring volume. Intellectual, yet not intellectualized, this book offers a comprehensive course of study in the challenges and opportunities of engaging in psychotherapeutic consultation with college students, a group whose utilization of psychological services has been steadily increasing over the past quarter century.

This scholarly yet accessible book will be essential reading for psychotherapy and college counseling trainees, early career professionals and senior clinicians, supervisors and administrators alike.'
Anton H. Hart, *FABP, FIPA*

'Rosenbaum and Webb have produced a remarkable work of scholarship. Drawing upon semiotics, existential philosophy, attachment theory, and Lacanian, interpersonal and relational psychoanalysis, they have woven together a highly sophisticated, but eminently readable, theoretical foundation upon which rests their understanding of psychotherapy as a collaborative and affirming undertaking through which therapists help patients uncover the "multitudes within" in order to live more authentic and fulfilled lives. The authors pay special attention to late adolescence and emerging adulthood, but in a refreshing departure from the familiar and easy logic of a rigid sequence of developmental steps toward the consolidation of identity, they offer instead a view of development as a richly textured, lifelong, and always incomplete journey. For all its erudition, this book is a also a highly pragmatic guide to addressing a range of challenging clinical problems, trauma and suicidal behaviors among them, sure to benefit even the most experienced

of therapists, and especially those working in college mental health settings. A true marvel!'
Richard J. Eichler, *Executive Director of Counseling & Psychological Services at Columbia University*

'Taking a fresh look at late adolescence and young adulthood, Philip Rosenbaum and Rick Webb address the core dynamic issues that emerge during this crucial developmental period. Using Lacan, Erikson, object relations and existential theories as a wide theoretical framework, they delineate the central issues with which therapists working with this population contend (constructive and destructive processes, suicide, trauma, relating to otherness, and tribalism).

Theoretically sophisticated, thoughtful, and scholarly, Rosenbaum and Webb move between the theoretical and the clinical, always retaining an overarching theoretical frame that allows the reader to discern the source(s) of the therapist's interventions. This book is a must read for clinicians working with this population'.
Joyce Slochower, *Professor Emerita of Psychology at Hunter College & the Graduate Center, CUNY; faculty, NYU Postdoctoral Program; author of* Holding and Psychoanalysis: A Relational Perspective *(1996, 2014)*

'Rick Webb and Phil Rosenbaum have given the world of counseling of college students an erudite and practically useful coverage of how psychoanalytic psychotherapy is not just a tool for treating different clinical cases but an ally that makes the guidance of student development possible. This is a rare focus in both psychoanalysis and in college level education—much needed as the future of the students is what matters most in the humanistic future of our Society.'
Jaan Valsiner, *Professor of Cultural Psychology, Aalborg University; Denmark Foreign Member, Estonian Academy of Sciences*

Contents

Acknowledgments

Getting to the point of writing the acknowledgments feels for me as a type of reward that is earned after a long journey. The acknowledgments are the place to reflect, offer thanks and appreciations for all those who in small or large ways participated in the creation of something that is special.

This book would not have come into existence without my being hired by Rick, while he was the Director of Counseling and Psychological Services at CAPS. So, it is here that I start. Having had few collaborators, I am sure that I am unaware of how fortunate I am that Rick and I get along as well as we do. Our conversations, disagreements and back and forth are almost always generative. More importantly, they are full of levity mixed with seriousness. It's been truly a joy to work with him not only on this book but our other articles as well and I look forward to what comes next.

My senior staff colleagues and friends at Haverford are certainly another reason that this book came into being. When I was hired by Rick, I did not know what I would inherit a family. This included Jane Widseth, Rebecca Ergas and Cynthia Guinyard. More recently, it has been expanded to Adam Edmunds, Pamela Lehman, Jon Krigel and Cameron O'Mara and most recently, Noël Shipp and Kaamila Mohamed. Each of these wonderful people has read articles, been subject to esoteric philosophical conversation and been a source of thoughtful dialogue and engagement. I am truly lucky to have such terrific colleagues and friends. Much in this book has been touched and influenced by them in small and large ways. Beyond senior staff, I am indebted to our trainees many of whom pose questions, engage in dialogue and stimulate meaningful conversation.

At Haverford, my work has been very well supported by any number of Deans and valued colleagues. I am particularly appreciative of the support provided by Dean Kelly Wilcox who not only puts with me but encourages me. Also of note are Dean's Martha Denney, Joyce Bylander, John McKnight, Katrina Glanzer and Steve Watter.

Special mention has to go to the students, some of whose stories are reflected in this book and many others who I have interacted with in numerous capacities over the years. It's tricky to write this type of book. I'm aware that in doing so I am in some ways using clinical material for my own self-advancement. It is my hope that this self-interest is buffeted by the ways that such writing helps me become a better clinician and so better able to treat others. Moreover, that other clinicians will read this book and that it may shift parts of their views to allow for more meaningful engagement with other patients as well.

Outside of Haverford, I have been lucky to be supported by an ever-growing personal and professional community. Special mention to my friend Ari Pizer. Our weekly talks and his willingness to read our writing have been both a source of ongoing stimulation and support and encouragement. Numerous other relationships, especially those associated with the William Alanson White Institute, are also reflected in the pages of this book. I am of course grateful to Donnel Stern for considering this book and welcoming it into his book series. My parents, Lee and Linda, sister Emily, brother-in-law Mike and babies Harrison and Caleb, as well as my in-laws Steve and Karen, have been and continue to be incredible sources of support.

As always, the most special thank you to my wonderful wife Michelle, who put up with my waking up early while writing. That she did so during a pandemic with a million and one other things going on is no small accomplishment. I am constantly amazed by her and am deeply appreciative of her. Lastly, this probably would not have been done without the love of my children Ethan and Julie. They have inspired me to consider development anew and afresh and are a source of surprise, joy and wonder. Thank you all.

Philip J. Rosenbaum

I benefit greatly from having family whose lively engagement with life has allowed them to grace me with the solitary space and peace of mind necessary to organize the meanderings of my mind into the words that contribute to this book. Thank you, Deb, my wife; Zack, Nate and Sam, our sons; and Tabitha, Ana and Tatiana, daughters-in-law. Their love nourishes me with the confidence to extend myself outward into the world because I know they will always welcome me home.

A soaring gratitude I also feel to Brennan, Ollie and Max, our grandsons. They bless Deb and me with the opportunity with them to tumble on the floor, negotiate nutrition, nap, discover bugs, throw rocks in the creek, watch cartoons while snacking, be superheroes that rescue, and, in general, express feelings and thoughts with unabashed honesty and enthusiasm. I missed a full appreciation of the complexity and beauty of awakening being-ness when our sons entered our lives. Getting a second chance at this is without comparison. It feeds my soul, and with my musings about it my intellect is stirred in ways no page of words can offer.

A heartfelt thanks to Kevin Cloherty, my buddy since first grade. Despite his conservatism, he lights me up with Irish wit. In his energetic difference from me, he also holds my feet to fire, challenging me to come to terms with my prejudices and assumptions. He will not read this book, and that is OK by me. It is more than enough that we reminisce our youth while we do home projects together in between getting pissed at each other for being stubborn. He's the essential buddy.

I am indebted to Philip in ways for which I cannot do justice. When Philip came to Haverford College, I knew within short order that with his intellectual openness, wisdom and sense of fairness he would carry CAPS forward with an abiding and deep appreciation of culture, the internal complexity of personhood, and the value of working hard. Our conversations over the past years always enrich my thoughts and stir new elaborations. I could not ask for a better writing partner. I hasten to add, however, that Philip joins a pantheon of colleagues and friends that have enriched my life. In addition to Haverford trainees whose astute questions demanded reasonable explanation or acknowledgment of ignorance, certain specific special persons rush from heart to mind: Ian Birky, David Bushnell, Cynthia Guinyard, Rebecca Ergas and Jane Widseth. These five set the pattern for the type of conversations I have with Philip, and they continue to be friends with whom I relish thinking about "things." I especially want to mention Jane, who as my predecessor as Director of CAPS, took a chance on hiring me and who, over more than 40 years, has alternately led me and accompanied me through the vagaries of many professional and life situations. She is a gem that life's serendipity sometimes affords us, a sister I never had.

Little of what is in this book could come about, of course, without the sharing of the people who have sought out my consultation over the years. They've changed my life immensely, and I cherish the opportunities I had to be invited into their worlds.

Lastly, my thanks to Donnell Stern for giving Philip and me this opportunity to express ourselves in print.

Richard E. Webb

Introduction

In this book, we hope to articulate, integrate and explore our ideas about working clinically with college-aged students in a college or university counseling center. We recognize, of course, that a person can be any age when attending college, but we are focusing on the "typically aged" student who falls within the range of 17–22 years of age. The student who enters college at the back end of adolescence and then in the course of his or her studies emerges into young adulthood. This is a fascinating developmental period. It is a time where individuals embrace and bear their way of being in the world, which often reshapes itself with marked changes.

Our intention is to provide a clinically based theory that has helped us make sense of and understand the complexity of these changes during this developmental period. To do this, we propose that our understanding of adolescence and young adulthood requires a sophisticated and nuanced theory that also considers the years leading up to this time in life. We think that much of the disconnect about adolescents these days reflects a problematic desire to simplify their experience or offer alienating contrasts with adolescents of other time periods. To address this, we try to offer a fresh look at the relevant developmental processes and to engage the complexity inherent to them. In doing this, we focus on numerous topics we think are pertinent to the life of the typically aged college student, but which are often, understandably, the source of confusion and consternation to older adults.

These include constructive and destructive processes (Chapter 4), suicide (Chapter 5), trauma and its effects (Chapter 6), relating to

DOI: 10.4324/9781003246558-1

otherness (Chapter 7) and tribalism (Chapter 8). We also include a chapter (Chapter 3) on clinical theory and technique, which is based on our developmental model and which we hope provides a broad understanding of how our theory informs practice. We do not specifically offer a chapter on emergent adolescent identity, peers and friend groups, and questions about agency. However, we recognize that these are important topics of consideration, and so we address them in our theoretical chapters (Chapters 1 and 2) and entwine our viewpoint on these topics throughout the book.

While we have written our topic-specific chapters to be accessible without directly engaging our theoretical sections (Chapters 1 and 2), we hope that the reader will start with chapters that lay out our theoretical foundations because we think this ultimately will provide the reader with a fuller appreciation of the complexity inherent to the topics of the subsequent chapters. Nevertheless, in the spirit of the non-linearity of adolescence, we try to allow for the reader to engage our book in their own fashion. Accordingly, we refer back and forth within the chapters to other chapters to try and link them together and to inform the reader's progression.

Who are Philip and Rick? Situating ourselves

As preface to our comments, we think it important to situate ourselves. Our thinking in this book primarily reflects our 50 years of cumulative, clinical experience as cis-gender heterosexual males working with students attending Haverford College: a small, liberal arts, co-educational institution with a Quaker heritage that is located in the suburbs of Philadelphia. Secondarily, it reflects experience we have garnered from the array of administrative relationships we have had both with students and with colleagues who are guiding these students' educational paths. Lastly, our ideas reflect our research endeavors both singularly and collaboratively.

Regarding our work together, we entered into conversation with each other with Rick being heavily influenced by Jacques Lacan, the existential philosophy of Sartre, and object-relations theorists, especially the writing of Thomas Ogden, and Donald Winnicott regarding developmental positions (i.e., autistic-contiguous, paranoid-schizoid, depressive and transcendent). Philip while also interested in existentialism has been influenced by his analytic training in interpersonal-relational thinking at the William Alanson White Institute and time spent studying cultural psychology before that. Writing together grew out of our lively discussions where we compared and contrasted different theories and how we thought these theories informed our clinical work, particularly as regards the topics we have chosen for chapters in this book.

We excitedly note that over the course of our collaboration our theoretical identities shifted as we found the courage to question our previously unchallenged ideas about what happens during early development/attachment. This, not surprisingly, coincides with Rick becoming a grandparent and Philip becoming a parent, not to mention the continuous evolution of attachment theory and relational writing. We acknowledge all this because we know that our experiences have been both constrained and embellished by our context and particular histories. As we will discuss at length throughout this manuscript, where our feet have been and where they rest both limit and enable the perceptual field. There can be no meaning-making and construction of experience without boundaries (Valsiner, 2009). Accordingly, we do our best to both note and explore how our location in the world greatly influences what we see and, therefore, how we evaluate it.

Any constraint, like any clinical experience, shapes our imperfect efforts to elaborate our understandings. Indeed, our recognition of this is an important reason for why we have organized our thoughts about doing psychotherapy with college-aged students for this book. Our systematic organization of what we have come to believe and understand allows opportunities for others to share their convergent and divergent perspectives. While we have theories and ideas about adolescence and young adults that we feel passionately about and believe worthy of consideration, we sincerely think that knowledge grows and refines itself through conversation with others.

Indeed, as we will discuss in the next section, part of the reason for co-authoring this book is to articulate how our individual perspectives have changed over the years through the rich dialogue we have had working collaboratively for more than five years. We view our theories and our applications of them to be thoughts in progress and hope that readers will engage them with similar spirit.

Why does adolescence feel insufficiently understood?

From our perspective, the developmental phase that pertains to late adolescence and young adulthood and characterizes most college-aged students remains an area that is insufficiently understood and sparsely attended to with theory (Kaplan, 1996). While widely recognized as a fungible time where great change can happen, fresh and evolving theories about the psychological processes underlying this period are hard to find. This is remarkable since this group draws national attention as one of the broadest and most financially engaged segments of our population. Furthermore, adolescents and young adults are oftentimes a great proportion of those who are the vanguard in protesting wars and in advocating for civil rights and social justice.

While a full review of adolescent development is outside the purview of this work, an overview of a few theories highlights prevailing trends. First, there is the enduring legacy of G. Stanley Hall who, in the early 20th century, characterizes adolescence as a period of *sturm und durg* (storm & strife) (Hall, 1904). He highlights idealism, ambitiousness, rebelliousness, passion and penchant for emotional turbulence. He notes how conflicts arise in the wash of seeing matters as critical one moment and then unimportant or forgotten a few moments later. While this view of adolescence captures the temperamental nature of this developmental period (Freud, 1958), we consider it not only unflattering but also problematic at times in that it casts adolescents and emerging adults as persons with delimited capacity for reason and, consequently, persons easily judged as beyond understanding and unavailable for productive interpersonal engagement. Hall's views easily lead to the quip that adolescents are creatures better locked away until the more settled hormone days of full adulthood are insured. Not surprisingly then, this has led to a host of theories which focus on how to manage adolescent conduct, and how to weather it with knowing smiles rather than engaging it as worthy because of its purposefulness and meaningfulness.

Erik Erikson's (1950) theory takes a more normative approach. He usefully focuses on emergent identity (we would now say "identities") and the various interpersonal crises that emerge during adolescence and lead to interpersonal conflict. So, a second trend, one that pivots from a normative framework, also views conflict as an essential part of adolescence. Acknowledgment and discussion of this make sense to us, but we will amplify how conflict is not just something to be weathered and survived but something fully to engage. Indeed, it is ironic that one of the virtues associated with adolescents, malleability and openness to change is something which often hinges on conflict. We are reminded and influenced by Heinz Werner's (1957) orthogenetic principle that articulates the view that for new differentiations to occur structures first have to de-differentiate. For something to change there often first has to be a receptivity to it. To recast anything such as metal or clay requires first that it lose something of its form. This is a theme to which we will return frequently in this book.

Erikson considered later adolescence to be a period of "psychosocial moratorium," an open space for trying on various ways of being and various identities without an essential commitment to them. Whether the openness of this space is (or was ever) as free as Erickson views is worthy of debate. In any case, we appreciate the idea embedded within this perspective that adolescents can function in various in-between and liminal spaces without solidifying the articulation of this functioning. Associated with this, it is worth noting that in much of contemporary culture there seems to be more tolerance for this moratorium, this suspension of commitment. Indeed, it is reasonable to say that adolescence has been extended into the ages of 18–25 years, a period now called "emerging adulthood" (Arnett, 2000). That this is so, of course, speaks to the socially constructed nature of adolescence and the risks of essentializing a particular period or developmental process.

When this occurs, and adolescents are seen as groups to be classified, categorized and essentially reified along lists "describing them"; rather than seen as engaging a lifelong journey of developmentally "becoming," it sets the stage for numerous valuations and judgments. Not surprisingly, especially when called millennials, adolescents are vulnerable to characterizations as entitled (Alton, 2017), less resilient (Larson, 2019; Gillespie 2019) and so forth. From our position as college clinicians, we frequently hear how adolescents of today, when compared to previous generations, are "sicker," more likely to experience "mental illness" (Lipson et al., 2021), less able to cope with normal stressors (like less than perfect academic grades)

(American Psychological Association, 2015), and more easily "triggered" by (vulnerably reactive to) communications and materials that might connote something aggressive or sexual (McQuade & Were, 2019). We think these kinds of judgments are often made with limited appreciation of the hand we all play in shaping the larger, cultural and social context that adolescents and emerging adults must adaptively negotiate. Without this appreciation, we are bewildered and confused by adolescents and emerging adults, and we falter in recognizing that they are agentic, meaning-making individuals who are entering in a forceful and lively way into the world of symbolism, naming, being, feeling and thinking.

We think the lagging understanding and consideration of this developmental period stems also from difficulty in appreciating and accommodating the paradoxes inherent to it. There are, of course, paradoxes inherent to any developmental period of living but those of college-aged students seem particularly challenging. These paradoxes are reflected by two main theories. One views adolescents as facing developmental challenges that are a recrudescence of those faced in childhood (Blos, 1962). This includes the challenges inherent to issues surrounding separation and individuation, rapprochement and trust. A second typical view, as noted earlier, is that adolescents are simply less rational and less settled versions of the full adults they almost are. They face concerns about intimacy and the difficulties entailed in coordinating a life path with a sense of one's own and other's capabilities, talents and opportunities. From the position of these two theoretical tendencies, this developmental period is seen as one in which meaning-making, relationship attachment, social awareness and intellectual exercise occur by beings who are either "big kids" or "little adults."

How this book addresses this insufficient understanding

Given that the relative uniqueness of this phase of development is usually not underlined and given its own status, we begin this book with theoretical and philosophical perspectives. We recognize that our level of abstraction might not be every reader's predilection, but we believe that efforts to engage the basic issues of adolescence and emerging adult life are rewarded most fruitfully with an overarching framework in place.

As we stated earlier, we do not consider adolescents and college-aged students to be understood fairly within a perspective that appoints their being-ness the simplified status of "big kid" or a "little adult." Instead, we view them as having a complexity that reflects a developmental period unique in its own way. That said, we hasten to say that college-aged students *are* dealing with existential-relational challenges that are relevant to us throughout our lifespan. Indeed, it is our interest and insistence on understanding development as a lifelong process that drives our clinical interest and which perhaps separates us from others who write about adolescence.

The uniqueness of adolescence: Immediacy and newness

What is unique to the developmental period of college-aged students and what gives it the sense of urgency and tempestuousness is the passionate immediacy that accompanies newness. In other words, a hallmark of adolescent experience is their grappling with these existential-relational challenges often for the first time with their feet standing so clearly alone in the world. The relative novelty of this provides them a fresh perspective which is less accessible to those who have already moved through it. Indeed, envy at not having this perspective or being denied it during our own adolescence may speak to some of the vitriol or idealization we afford those of this developmental period. As writer Joseph Conrad long ago wistfully mused: "I remember my youth and the feeling that will never come back anymore – the feeling that I could last forever, outlast the sea, the earth and all men" (1898/2021, unnumbered).

This newness and immediacy, always constrained by context and space, of course, gives adolescence and emerging adulthood its uniqueness, sense of possibility and well-worn challenges. This is also what makes college-aged students more vulnerable to being overwhelmed, carried away or reactive to these challenges. This brings with it "good" and the "bad." On the one hand, adolescents can be less tolerant of certain political maneuvers or truisms; they come into awareness about otherness with tremendous energy and need for change (Webb & Rosenbaum, 2021). Similarly, they can be less jaded or cynical about the possibilities of change, more convinced that simple but firm resolve "to do" will be sufficient for achieving success.

Their delimited experience in life can mean that they experience the "no's" or the frustrations of life with not only more immediacy but also with more passionate expectation, hopeful or otherwise, than we adults who have more history with disappointment and success. We hasten to add that working with adolescents and emerging adults becomes incredibly enriching when we respectfully can remember and locate them within our own developmental arc and thereby hold them as the link not only to our own past but also to our future. It provides an opportunity to reconsider continually our own histories of being and a way of keeping us as therapists young at heart. This is a clinical sensibility we strongly endorse throughout this book.

Some important considerations

Before moving on we want to note the conundrum of how language does not always capture our emergent sensitivities about diversity, equity and social justice. Although language is always alive and evolving, there is often not a comfortable way within it both to acknowledge historical tradition and yet not be bound by the precedent of it.

Throughout the book, we use he/him language for self-identification. We recognize that this may be problematic to some more than others and that there are a variety of ways to address questions of who is reading and who is writing. We have chosen to use this language not as a default but as an important way of recognizing our own situated-ness and as a way of keeping our own gender in mind with respect to how it influences our perspective.

We also frequently talk about relational constellations that have roots in early parent-child dynamics. For example, Chapter 1 focuses upon our discontinuity following our emergence from our symbiotic relationship with our primary caretaker. In the literature, this person is almost always referred to as "mother." In Chapter 2, we focus more on the need to de-authorize our caregiver who is often thought of as "father." In our work, we are continually searching for a manageable way to express that these roles can be filled by people irrespective of their biology, sex, or gender. Where we have currently landed is first to note and describe the role being performed at a particular developmental junction. We then refer to the person playing this role as either

M-other or *F-other*. In doing so, we try to nod to the traditional denotation that has saturated literature, while simultaneously acknowledging that the occupation of these roles is not dictated by conventional designation. We ask for the reader's grace in working with us to look for the element of truth that we pursue even if our language fails to capture it. (Does it, language, ever capture it?)

With respect to how we refer to developmental positions, we go back and forth about whether to keep to the original names: autistic-contiguous, paranoid-schizoid, depressive and transcendent. The two middle names were originally conceived by Melanie Klein (1975a, 1975b), and the first and last were largely formalized by Thomas Ogden (1986, 1989) and James Grotstein (2007). Indeed, elsewhere (Webb & Rosenbaum 2021) we have simply referred to these positions in an ordinal way: first, second and so forth. This is an idea which we adopted while thinking of dance, yoga and other pursuits of movement. Movement, of course, is relevant since these positions importantly reflect how we occupy space in the world.

We realize that the original names might be off-putting, but they are ones that, of course, have evolved over time and in the throes of the politics that can underlie the evolution of theory in any field. That said, meaning-making is never stagnant, and sometimes modification of terminology is warranted. We recognize that current sensitivities rightfully encourage a perspective that associates autism with a segment of persons who are different from the neurotypical community. Hence, hereafter, we refer to the first position noted earlier as simply the "contiguous" position.

The issue of how these positions should be named is not new. Here's a brief story shared by British psychoanalyst, John Padel:

> I remember a scientific meeting of c.1955 at which Winnicott regretted the common use of the term of 'The Depressive Position' rather than, say, 'the stage of concern,' but decided that it had come to stay, so he would accept and use it himself; but he couldn't accept the 'paranoid-schizoid position' as an account of the baby's earliest weeks of life. When Klein got up, she said she'd waited 20 years for Dr Winnicott to accept her term 'depressive position' and she could wait another 20 to hear him accept the 'paranoid-schizoid position'. (1989, p. 2)

While keeping these names might be seen as putting new wine in old bottles (Orange, 2011), we prefer to think of how spirits aged in old wine casks blend different chemistries to create richer body. We think this analogy is especially apt because it alludes to the complexity that underlies the phenomenological complexion of these positions.

Lastly, throughout the book, we refer to our patients as a mixture of patients and clients. While consistency for the sake of consistency would be nice, we each think of them differently and so try and hold to both ways. When appropriate we use case material to help illustrate our ideas. When possible, we have sought permission from student-patients. However, given the long scope of our practice, this hasn't always been feasible.

We, in any case, go to great lengths to disguise our student-clients so as to ensure their confidentiality, including at times creating composite cases that are based upon our individual clinical work and also our ongoing supervision of trainees. Accordingly, we have decided to keep the voice of the therapist in the third person rather than the more personal and subjective identification. While this is against the grain of how we view ourselves as practicing and the theoretical and clinical orientation we value, it also helps respect confidentiality and the varied nature of our practice and source of clinical information. Moreover, we think it reads a bit more fluidly rather than trying to introduce ourselves as the clinician. We hope that readers bear with us in this more impersonal presentation of ourselves.

Overview of the book

By way of broad sweep, this book is organized first by theory and then by offering a more phenomenological and close-at-hand read of how we emerge as subjects. As the chapters progress, so too does our perspective, such that by the end we have "zoomed out" to consider how and why we organize into groups (or tribes). Notably, we hold throughout the book the dynamic tension between self and other by which we are both becoming articulated and possibly undifferentiated. Our focus and organization on first the phenomenology and then the broader culture perhaps reflects our thinking as clinicians and stems out of our pivot from developmental and existential theory in Chapters 1 and 2 toward clinical practice in Chapter 3. We note, however, that self and other are mutually constitutive; so we cannot consider one without the other.

In Chapter 1, we discuss the consequences of our emergence out of symbiotic one-ness, first biologically from our mother and then psychologically from primary caregivers. In this separation-individuation process, we are disposed, with differing levels of awareness, to seek both our ongoing continuity with others, which is a return to a semblance of symbiosis, *and* our discontinuity or differentiation from others. This process involves our engagement with cultural structures of meaning-making. Hence, we discuss the importance of semiotics and of a cultural psychological approach to development that emphasizes the ways our ideas always stand in dynamic tension with one another.

In Chapter 2, we turn from discussing *what we are* to the question of *how we become* something with this *what*. This involves understanding how we become able to experience, tolerate and hopefully embrace others' differences, including the ways we are other or different from ourselves. We propose that this relationship to otherness pertains centrally to our pursuit of self-agency and authorization. We track this developmental progression and discuss at the end of the chapter some of what can go wrong.

In Chapter 3, we discuss the implications of Chapters 1 and 2 for the clinical theory and technique that informs our interventions throughout the book. While we at times may talk in the language of "knowing," we hope that the reader will understand that we are offering ideas to *stir* the pot of clinical thinking rather than to offer a defined recipe. Indeed, as our theory evolves so to does our understanding of what makes for "good" technique.

In Chapter 4, we begin to apply our thinking toward processes by which adolescents both create and destroy in their processes of becoming. While these processes sometimes involve literal actions, our focus is more upon the relational processes wherein *becoming* intrinsically and always entails *undoing* who we are. This, of course, sometimes involves also undoing or destroying how other people see us and we see them. In this chapter, we argue that these destructive processes have been too often located in early development and that they can better be appreciated in adolescence. Not only does this alleviate some of the potential challenges around thinking about childhood but also we think it helps further and ground our thinking about adolescent *becoming*.

In Chapter 5, our exposition of these processes in some ways continues with more of a focus on what can happen when the key others in our life are unable to tolerate our emergent subjectivity. We describe in detail how at the extreme end of this, suicidal crises can develop out of our relational need to *become* when our primary caregivers are significantly conflicted about our doing so. We describe relational impasses that lead us to view suicide as an option which both "solves" the problem and communicates the problem so that development might have a chance to move forward. In this, we emphasize the clinical need to create and sustain relationships with these patients.

In Chapter 6, we discuss trauma. As we did in Chapter 5, we again take up challenges in attachment, but we do so in less broad terms. We consider how more discrete and external events can impact our developing sense of self. To accomplish this, we build off contemporary views that hypothesize that our sense of "ourselves" is always multiple, fractured and relational. This provides us the basis by which we can look at the emergence of self in a micro-analytic way so that we can highlight the dual processes of dissociation and enactment. We discuss at length these normative processes before exploring their role when we become traumatized. Finally, we talk about the treatment of trauma within the "fishbowls" of our university and college contexts and note some of the opportunities and challenges this unique context provides.

Our focus on Chapter 7 broadens to include more consideration about the importance of otherness for our developing sense of self and the challenges that this can entail in higher education. We describe how it is in our embrace (or not) of our relational need for the other, and they for us, that we become able to actualize ourselves in agentic and purposeful fashion. Notably, this entails a capacity to learn and be curious about the ways we are other to ourselves as well as other to others. In this, we appreciate that our need and desire to connect with others not only shores up our sense of being but also perhaps threatens it. In our relationships with difference, we have to be open to the process of being "unnamed" so as to rename. We discuss how contexts of higher education ambivalently facilitate this.

On the one hand, these contexts extoll the virtue of this but at other times myopically serve to forestall this dynamic process.

Finally, in Chapter 8, we zoom out to consider how and why we may organize ourselves into "tribes" or groups. This enables us to consider a serious question about our developmental theory and, more generally, about development and being. We consider what happens when in call to meaningful action we can stagnate in, lose or decide to change the existential-relational position in which we have been functioning? This question frequently comes up in our work with adolescents who are working to consolidate their nuanced views of self and other but struggling with the real harms, challenges and problems in the physical world. That these often seem to necessitate a firm and uncompromising response can lead to questions about the value and need of perspective. It is, perhaps, a mark of our relative privilege to be able to advocate for developmental nuance and complexity in the face of real systemic and societal oppressions. Nonetheless, we see important value in considering how we negotiate "groupal" type thinking (Gonzalez, 2016). Such consideration helps ground our actions, and it offers to us the always-welcome opportunity to be better able to choose how we affiliate in groups and respond to tribal thinking.

By way of the last word, we recognize that not everyone may share our zest for theory and philosophy, but we hope, at the very least, that our writing is able to capture some of the excitement we experienced in our collaboration both before and during this project. In this, we welcome dialogue and engagement. We can only hope for the continual conversation that has shaped and changed these ideas over the many years and the unknown surprise of where such discussion may land us with our thinking about self, adolescence, clinical work and developmental process.

References

Alton, L (2017, November 22). *Millennials and entitlement in the workplace: The good, the bad, and the ugly.* https://www.forbes.com/sites/larryalton/2017/11/22/millennials-and-entitlement-in-the-workplace-the-good-the-bad-and-the-ugly/?sh=28fbd7573943

American Psychological Association (2015). Stress in America: Paying with our health. https://www.apa.org/news/press/releases/stress/2014/stress-report.pdf.

Arnett, J (2000). Emerging adulthood: A theory of development from chelate teens through the twenties. *American Psychologist, 55* (5), 469–480. 10.1.1.462.7685. doi:10.1037/0003-066X.55.5.469.

Blos, P (1962). *On Adolescence, A psychoanalytic Interpretation.* The Free Press of Glencoe.

Conrad, J (2021, February 17). *Youth.* https://www.gutenberg.org/files/525/525-h/525-h.htm (Original work published 1898). This eBook is for the use of anyone anywhere in the United States and most other parts of the world at no cost and with almost no restrictions whatsoever. You may copy it, give it away or re-use it under the terms of the Project Gutenberg License included with this eBook or online at www.gutenberg.org.

Erikson, E (1950). *Childhood and society.* W.W. Norton.

Freud, A (1958). Adolescence. *The Psychoanalytic Study of the Child, 13* (1), 255–278. 10.1080/00797308.1958.11823182.

Gillespie, D (2019). *Teen Brain.* Sydney, Australia: MacMillan.

Gonzalez, F (2016). On the relation to non-relationality. *Psychoanalytic Dialogues, 26* (5), 522–531. 10.1080/10481889909539308.

Grotstein, JS (2007). *A beam of intense darkness, Wilfred Bion's legacy to psychoanalysis.* Karnac Press.

Hall, GS (1904). *Adolescence: Its psychology and its relation to physiology, anthropology, sociology, sex, crime, religion, and education* (Vols. 1 & 2). Prentice-Hall.

Kaplan, L (1996). The stepchild of psychoanalysis, Adolescence. *American Imago, 53* (3), 257–268. 10.1353/aim.1996.0008.

Klein, M (1975a). *The collected works of Melanie Klein, Volume I, love, guilt and reparation and other works 1921–1945.* The Free Press.

Klein, M (1975b). *The collected works of Melanie Klein, Volume III, envy, gratitude and other works 1946–1963.* The Free Press.

Larson, D (2019, May 6). Younger generations' lack of resiliency raises concerns for all ages. St. Cloud Times. Retrieved December 24, 2021, from https://www.sctimes.com/story/opinion/2019/05/03/younger-generations-lack-resiliency-raises-concerns-all-ages-millennials-generation-z/3662670002/

Lipson SK, Phillips, MV, Winquist, N, Eisenberg, D, Lattie, EG (2021). Mental health conditions among community college students: A national study of prevalence and use of treatment services. *Psychiatric Services,* appi.ps.2020004. 10.1176/appi.ps.202000437.

McQuade, K, & Were., T (2019, August 22). *What the 'snowflake generation' understands about trauma.* https://time.com/5659268/trigger-warnings-snowflake-generation/.

Ogden, TH (1986). *The matrix of the mind, Object relations and the psychoanalytic dialogue*. Jason Aronson.

Ogden, TH (1989). *The Primitive edge of experience*. Jason Aronson.

Orange, DM (2011). *The suffering strange: Hermeneutics for everyday clinical practice*. Routledge.

Padel, J (1989, March 10). *The psychoanalytical theories of Melanie Klein and Donald Winnicott and their interaction in the British Society of Psychoanalysis* [Paper presentation]. Philadelphia Society for Psychoanalytic Psychology, Spring Meeting.

Valsiner, J (2009). Cultural psychology today: Innovations and oversights. *Culture & Psychology*, *15* (1), 5–39. 10.1177/1354067x08101427.

Webb, RE & Rosenbaum, P (2021). Embracing diversity: The complexities of reckoning and accepting otherness. *Integrative Psychological and Behavioral Science*, *50* (1), 30–46. DOI: 10.1007/s12124-020-09582-9.

Werner, H (1957). The concept of development from a comparative and organismic point of view. In D Harris (Ed.), *The concept of development, An issue in the study of human behavior* (pp. 125–148). University of Minnesota Press.

Chapter 1

Important Aspects of Our Existential Nature and Meaning-Making

We feel that our thinking about college and university students has to begin with considering the ontological aspect of our (and their) existential-relational condition. In other words, before moving to discuss periods, phases and phenomena of development specific to young adulthood, we have to reflect on our fundamental nature as beings. Indeed, while consideration of this is relevant throughout all of our lifespans, from our perspective it takes on significant urgency during the college years of late adolescent and young adults. Hence, before we can address the various ways, we progressively and alternately organize the particulars of "what we are," we must appreciate "who we are."

In our approach to addressing the question of "being," we consider two aspects of our existential-relational situation that are common to all of us:

1 The tension between continuity and discontinuity that is intrinsic to our sense of being-ness as we emerge out of symbiotic one-ness with our primary caretaker and face the challenge of how to separate and individuate ourselves from others while also maintaining our connection to them.
2 How we make meaning out of our life experiences through our essential reliance on the acquisition and use of semiotic (sign) systems which are always culturally experienced before being internalized.

DOI: 10.4324/9781003246558-2

Finding continuity/discontinuity in our being in relation to difference

Some problems with the usual state of "separation and individuation"

Our emergence into the world starts with our separation away from our symbiotic one-ness with our primary caregiver. While usually referred to as "mother," we note that this can be any primary care-giver whose role is central to our well-being and to create "good enough" conditions for us to be safe and to flourish (Winnicott, 1971). As stated in our introduction, in acknowledgment of this caregiver's non-specific gender, we, hereafter, will refer to this person either as a primary caregiver or as "M-other." In any case, this person is ideally one who is invested in our care and who provides sufficient conditions for us to emerge as an agentic being.

Not surprisingly, much of developmental literature rightfully focuses on the process of "separation/individuation," with numerous books having been devoted to this natural process (Mahler et al., 1975/2000). Usually, this literature maps out the stages that can be identified as we proceed from infancy to childhood and then on through adolescence to separate or individuate from our family and our assortment of key caregivers. While we think the idea of separation/individuation is important, we find the typical ways of dealing with this process insufficient for two reasons.

First, they often fail to note how this is an ongoing and lifelong process. Indeed, Erik Erikson (1950) is one of the few clinical the-orists whose "staging" acknowledges this. However, we propose that the staging, especially past adolescence, is not robust. Second, per-haps even more importantly, we maintain that even when these stages are loosely applied, our existential nature is misrepresented or over-looked. Characteristically, stage theories imply a subjective teleology that there is an endpoint toward which all the stages march. In as much as this is so, most developmental theories do not acknowledge that an essential aspect of our being-ness is our incompletion even as we proceed toward greater differentiation.

Continuity/discontinuity and completion/incompletion

We suggest that a worthy alternative approach is one that captures the dynamic interplay in our being-ness between seeking completion/

continuity and incompletion/discontinuity. A theory is needed that appreciates our ontological condition and that thereby is able to highlight the tension between our search for a coherence in *and* evolution of who we are to ourselves and others. The psychoanalyst, Jacques Lacan, is pertinent in this regard. He (1977) considers how our march into and through iterations of being-ness is an intrinsically challenging one, which starts with the physical rupture of the symbiotic relationship the mother and child share while the child is in the womb and then proceeds immediately into the psychological realm where it is played out in our connection and individuation from important others in our life. Lacan sees this original separation as alienating to the child since the child only is able to construct an image (identity) of themselves through the fragmented perspectives of their caretakers. Only being able to glimpse ourselves through these fragmented reflections of our caregivers' perceptions means that our experience of ourselves, especially during our early years, is known to us fundamentally in the refracted way that characterizes our socially constructed identity.

This process engenders an elusiveness of identity in any essential sense. We come to experience and so know, who we are through the gaze of important others in our lives, as well as our broader society and culture. Hence, our sense of "being" and of who we are, is always plural, multiple and reflective of our numerous relationships. Within this complex plurality of images and refractions, we search continually to find a coherence within which we can distinguish boundaries between ourselves and others and therein articulate identities, which feel specific and authentic to our own being.

Lacan further notes that it is not adequate to speak of "an identity" only in relation to others. Our identity also speaks to who we are in relation to ourselves. In other words, our sense of ourselves emerges not only out of our relationship to others but also out of our experience and understanding of who we are to our own self. Assuming we do not contravene the nature of our ontology by deluding ourselves into thinking that this journey can end prior to our death, we must embrace the idea that our identity is always something that is in pursuit of itself. We are always "becoming." As Mikkel Borch-Jacobsen says,

For Lacan, it would no longer be a question of recognizing one's self in the mirror; on the contrary, the issue would be *not* to recognize oneself in the mirror, to shatter it and move on, bloodied, into the void of its absence. (1991, p. 81)

Our incompletion, then, is what constitutes our existential condition. It is both our lifelong challenge and our potential for the pleasure of ongoing newness. "[W]here the real journey begins" is beyond "the ecstatic limit of *'Thou are that'*" (Lacan, 1977, p. 7, original emphasis).[1] We and others can only frame our sense of our being within the realm of words and cultural understandings, but the fact is that this is so means that our reference point for being "named" is always one that can claim no relationship with an unfiltered reality. In short, our identity is something that can never be fully captured by any construction of meaning available to us within the ever-changing relativity of culture and words. Therefore, it is something, as we noted earlier, which we can ever view as complete. As Jacques Lacan says, "There is nowhere any last word unless in the sense in which *word* is *not a word* ... Meaning indicates the direction in which it fails" (1982, p. 150, original emphasis). Gary Whitehead says in his poem, *A Glossary of Chickens*, we should not assume, "that by naming we can understand,/as if the tongue were more than muscle" (2010, p. 39). The "should" in this is something we will shortly discuss when we focus on the completion/incompletion nuance within continuity/discontinuity.

As such, our identity is not something which should not be considered a stable "achievement" but rather as something which is always in the process of developing and becoming. Keys to navigating this shifting world of identities are the ways that we come to experience ourselves as individuals who have and bear responsibility for our own desires and the capacities to pursue these desires. The attachment theorists (Beebe, 2005; Beebe & Lachmann, 1998, 2003, 2014; Beebe et al., 2012; Stern, 1983; Schore & Schore, 2008) highlight how the bi-directional and mutually regulating relationships between babies and their caregivers set the stage for our emergent multiplicities and agency. In this regard, they extend beyond Lacan's understanding of rupture and alienation toward articulation of the challenging and complicated relational factors that are at play. As the burgeoning child, we experience not only positive attachment with our caregivers but ambivalence. Always present is the potential for an attachment that reflects avoidance or disorganization. Our caregivers attach to us in a corresponding way, and the complex mix of factors mentioned above is especially in play when our caregivers have experienced trauma. However, as we will discuss later, the potential for dysregulation in the attachment is present when, for whatever reason, conditions are not "good enough."

Operating from this perspective which acknowledges our ontological state means that there is no "endpoint" to our efforts to distinguish ourselves with identities. Our nature is not a march toward some ultimate state of organized identity but rather a journey, within the embrace of our continuity with others, always to express our discontinuity, "the cipher of [our] mortal destiny" (Lacan, 1977, p. 7). The choice of the terms continuity/discontinuity and completion/incompletion, then, is our effort to undermine any notion that we are proceeding to some ultimate existential state of definition. Notably, as we will discuss more in the next chapter, this process can be thwarted in numerous ways and, indeed, much of our work as clinicians involve navigating these situations.

An alternative metaphor: Articulation and collapse

In considering the processes related to continuity and discontinuity, we have found ourselves drawn away from the confines of psychology toward borrowing a concept from quantum physics which we think serves well as a metaphor, as a way of thinking of how we, as beings, are disposed to exist within our worlds (Rosenbaum & Webb, 2021). In doing this, we are in some ways appreciating the efforts behind apophatic or negative theology, a speaking toward what is always beyond words by "speaking away" (Webb & Sells, 1995).

In quantum physics, the subatomic matter is viewed as having a duality in its nature. Such matter is simultaneously a wave and a particle. A "gaggle" of matter travels as wave which is everywhere and nowhere at the same time. It has, however, a potentiality to manifest when it "collapses" into a particle, into matter with a particularized location. This happens when the gaggle of matter is observed or measured. Although collapsed in a given instance of observation, the matter that constitutes the particle continues to bring its duality into next events with the potential for new collapses into different particularizations.[2]

The dialectic between measurement and collapse is useful for meeting the challenges in describing how a person emerges into an interpersonally distinguishable being. From our perspective, we, as people, come into the world also as a gaggle of matter: we start our lives with a broad wave of potential self-states and identities. Over time, our potential delimits itself as we are measured or positioned in language by ourselves and others within our shared cultures. The process of being measured or named by others and ourselves within the fold of our culture's description of reality and the process of being freed from that measuring through recognition of culture's relativity is the movement back and forth between wave and particle. It is the movement which provides a complex backdrop for our emergent identities. It is a back and forth which entails the serial collapse of our being into articulation by naming and then our return to status as a "wave" of not-yet-named potential.

Of course, the use of metaphor to describe the dialectic of our being-ness is something others have also used. While we think quantum physics offers an especially useful means for capturing the process of articulation and then immersion in a one-ness, we wish to note, by contrast, how Friedrich Nietzsche has approached this same issue. To do this we rely particularly on Steven Mitchell's (1986) commentary on Nietzsche.

Nietzsche addresses the dialectic through the anchor of early Greek gods: Apollo, the god of dreams and illusion, and Dionysus, the god, who in an early version represents undoing and the death of the individual. In his theory of tragedy (1910/1872), Nietzsche heralds the "tragic man" who lives with and between both dimensions of being that are represented by these gods: (a) an Apollonian one wherein we emerge temporarily in some form of identity or articulation and (b) a Dionysian one wherein we dissolve into the undifferentiated oneness of "a larger unity, a universal pool of energy" (Mitchell, 1986, p. 195).

To explain Nietzsche's ideas about this, Steven Mitchell (1986) pictures the beach at low tide. He says that the Apollonian person builds castles out of sand with a fervor that bespeaks expectation that they will last forever, with passion that is oblivious to the inevitable destruction that the tide will bring. By contrast, the Dionysian person, Mitchell says, understands the ocean's rhythm and power and therefore forbears from any creation. Nietzsche's "tragic man" embodies the inclinations of both these gods, and Mitchell says that this person is "aware of the tide and the transitory nature of his productions, yet [builds] his sandcastles nevertheless" (p. 195), thus allowing for a rich, "dialectical interplay of illusion and reality" (p. 195).

Semiotic sign systems as a basis for meaning-making

While metaphor is important to help us hold in imagination complicated ideas, we must not overlook the importance of diving into theory, even if it is a complex endeavor. In this regard, a theorist of key importance is the pragmatist Charles S. Peirce. We will focus a good bit now on some of his ideas because we will later refer to them in summary ways when we turn our focus more particularly in the next chapter to toward named, developmental positions. As we discuss Peirce (1965), we will bridge his ideas to others, such as Lacan.

Peirce offers us theory which pertains to how we engage in meaning-making and how meaning-making depends centrally on a dialectic of continuity/discontinuity, completion/incompletion. To do this, Peirce describes semiosis, the process of using and creating signs (which includes words and all other forms of cultural symbols) to regulate or mediate our relationships within our environments. This mediation occurs at all levels of immediacy and abstraction, and it regulates, accordingly, how we relate to everything and everyone, including ourselves, within our environment.

Central to Peirce's ideas about semiotic mediation is that it is triadic rather than dyadic. Peirce describes a semiotic triangle composed of an object, a representamen and an interpretant. In his words:

A sign … [or representamen] is something which stands to somebody for something in some respect or capacity. It addresses somebody, that is, creates in the mind of that person an equivalent sign, or perhaps a more developed sign. That sign which it creates I call the interpretant of the first sign. The sign stands for something it's object. It stands for that object, not in all respects, but in reference to a sort of idea, which I have sometimes called the ground of the representamen. (1965, *V. 2*, p. 228)

Breaking this down, a sign is comprised of three parts that all relate to one another in particular ways. Peirce uses the word "sign" to refer to both the whole of the three parts and also a specific part that he terms the *representamen*. We will use this latter word despite it being a bit ungainly.

The *representamen* represents some aspect of an object to someone or something. The person's understanding or interpretation of what is being represented is termed by Peirce the *interpretant*. For our purposes, this *interpretant* can be viewed an equivalent of a more developed sign or as an interpretation of the object that is being represented. This interpretation can then itself become the object, which is then represented to either us or someone else. Peirce calls the ongoing nature of signification *semiosis*. While semiosis may be ongoing, it is importantly also constrained or limited by the ground of the representamen, which is the context where semiosis takes place. A sign as a whole then stands for some things but not all things. This means that semiosis or ongoing signification is ongoing and incomplete.

Peirce elaborated numerous categories of sign relationships or the ways that the different parts of the sign relate to each other. His three most famous are *icon, index and symbol.* An icon is when the representamen shares a resemblance with its object. Hence, a photograph is an iconic sign. An index is when there is a physical connection between object and representamen in the way that smoke indicates fire or a bullet hole indicates the bullet. Lastly, a symbol is when object and representamen are connected conventionally. This, then, encompasses words and language, which are conventional. Signs can be multiple things, so a photograph is not only iconic but perhaps also a symbol. Since signification occurs within the context of a ground, possible meanings shift such that a bullet hole looks very different on a billboard depending on whether its presence accompanies the advertisement of a store or a battlefield.

As humans, we are socialized from our earliest days into various sign systems such that our processes of making meaning and constructing experience are based on social and cultural convention. This is not only clear from Peirce's consideration that language is a symbolic and, as such, a conventional sign system but also his insistence upon the ground or the context where semiosis is taking place. This forces us to consider where we are physically and psychically situated when considering not only our own interpretation of events but also that of others.

This triangular system stands in contrast to the dyadic systems, such as that of de Saussure (2006/2002) which presupposes two parts: the signified and a signifier. These can be mapped onto Peirce's system as the object (signified) and the representamen (signifier). However, the dyadic account does not consider the role of the interpretant, i.e., that signified/signifier only take meaning in addressing someone (or something). Moreover, they are acontextual; they are devoid of ground and context. While this was not a problem for de Saussure (2006/2002) who intentionally was not developing a theory of psychological meaning-making (Rosa, 2007), it is a problem for its application into psychological processes. While stripping signified and signifier of context may allow for deconstruction of text and of narrative, it does so in ways that are not grounded and ultimately divorced from reality. This may have used in considering the ways that these relationships are arbitrarily constructed, it does not, from our perspective, provide a compelling account of how meaning develops. For this, we need a triadic theory that considers both interpretants (others) and context (ground).

Indeed, while not as explicitly integrated into psychoanalytic theory and practice as de Saussure, whose ideas are acknowledged by Lacan as important to his own,[3] we think that one of the core implicit tenets of the relational school in psychoanalysis is an unstated turn to triadic systems of meaning-making. Speaking to this, the interpersonal psychoanalyst, Edgar Levenson, describes psychoanalysis as a "circumscribed *semiotic event*" that involves "the transmission of signals, signs, signifiers and symbols in any communication system whatever" (1981, p. 496).

Notably, while Lacan draws more explicitly from the dyadic perspective of de Saussure (to the extent where it is a shortcoming of his clinical theory), we do think that Lacan shows a remarkable implicit understanding of the triadic perspective as reflected, for instance, in his considering of real, imaginary and symbolic. This is not surprising given his likely awareness of Peirce, but it would not have been keeping within his own ground to emphasize context and the inter-psychic beyond the intra-psychic. Since we maintain that this triadic perspective does not make its way into his clinical theory in satisfying ways especially as it pertains to our central focus on development, we work to add it in throughout the book in ways that we feel make sense to us and are consistent with our own personal readings of Lacan.

Theories of development: Dyadic versus triadic systems

In contrasting dyadic and triadic theories of meaning-making, Luca Tateo notes that "dyadic relationships never lead to development" (2016, p. 434). This is because dyads organize around poles of op-posing meaning. For example, in psychology there are ideas of nature versus nurture, collective versus individualistic and normative versus pathological. In psychoanalysis, there are inner versus outer, phan-tasy versus reality, surface versus depth and so forth. While these poles provide a certain clarification, they are ultimately recursive.

This is because they overly constrict the poles or ends of the field such that new meanings are essentially blocked. When we look to re-place one set of meanings with a pre-determined symbolic set of other meanings, i.e., when we argue outer versus inner, real versus phantasy, we actually block or obstruct the development of meaning. We hinder the natural process of allowing new continuity to emerge out of an embrace of discontinuity.

Returning to Levenson (2003), we might say that our me-tapsychology's dictate our meaning-making, such that during a ses-sion "one listens and then – out of a need to be useful – tries to figure out what it might mean" (p. 240). When we can resist the urge to make meaning and so stay below the plane, an imaginary horizon where data are either more abstract and organized or deconstructed and extended, we are in effect creating a triangle which allows ap-preciation of the vast network of meanings which might pertain or be relevant.

Stated somewhat differently, there is a pull to "be useful" and so "to know." This means applying metapsychological meaning into the field in a dyadic way, such as to describe the relationship between signifier/signified. When we can resist this pull toward a point-to-point system (x means y), we are able to create a triangle by which we can say something more like x means y (but also may mean w, v, ...) to z. Thus, we keep perspective and work to broaden signification. We are appreciating, in other words, that the "tongue" is "mere muscle," and we are taking a position which does not collapse the "wave of potential being" through an assumption that our voice has privileged authority to "measure."

Stuart Schneiderman (1990) captures the understanding of this in remarking on Lacan's view of the symptom as a function of stagnant meaning. Schneiderman writes,

> [Lacan] declares that the cutting edge of psychoanalytic inter-pretation is equivocation ... . The symptom is kept in place, is nourished and sustained by the belief that words maintain a singular relationship to meanings ... . The function of equivoca-tion is to subvert treatment, to institute a break between subject and symptom, and thus to permit the symptom's wording to rediscover the discourse it was part of before it was misappro-priated by the subject. (pp. 219–220)

We see the effects of dyadic systems throughout the psychoanalytic and psychological literature. Speaking to this, Levenson (1981) notes that "Intrapsychic analysis has affirmed such a stance and even the current literature is replete with clinical examples wherein the most blatant reality is ignored in pursuit of symbolization" (p. 491). Thus, the analyst is seen as possessing a clearer reality which they put over the patient's semiotic expression in effect substituting their ideas for the patients.

For example, in a more recent paper on depression by Charles Brenner (1991), he writes of a young woman's depression. Specifically, he says,

> The patient was a thirty-three-year-old unmarried woman who came for treatment complaining that she felt unhappy and did

not know what she wanted to do in life. Nothing seemed to interest her, she said. She had worked in her family's business for several years and had at first enjoyed being there, but she finally grew to dislike it and left. Since that time she had been at loose ends. (p. 38)

In considering the etiology of her depression, Brenner writes,

Nor was the onset of her symptoms difficult to discern. It coincided with the entry of her brother into family business. Until that time the patient had been he father's right hand in the business. When her brother, who was five years her junior and her only sibling, came into the business, it soon became clear to the patient that it was not she, but her brother, who was destined to be her father's close associate and eventual successor. It was then that her symptoms began. (p. 39)

Brenner's explanation of this is that the

Patient's conflicts centered about the fact that she was a girl, not a boy, and that they had done so since her brother's birth. Her penis envy and her misery at having been born a girl, which to her as a child meant having been castrated, were intense. (p. 39)

As readers of this case story, we must acknowledge that the nuanced understanding that emerges between a therapist and a patient within the intimacy of the consulting space is not something which can be fully conveyed in any written account. Nonetheless, Brenner's conclusion about his patient's conflict invites us at least to wonder if it reflects an entrenched dyadic view where analytic meta-theory, whether about Oedipal dynamics or early object relations, pre-determines the meanings of the field. When this happens, as we try to make clear above, this flattens "essentially" the field and impedes more authentic collaboration and co-construction around meaning.

Brenner, for instance, gives us no indication that he considered with his patient the reality of her being unceremoniously replaced by her brother who was five years her junior and who had a position bestowed upon him for which he was not as experientially qualified as she was. He does not explore competition, whether the woman felt oppressed or attacked. Thus, we think it reasonable to pose whether Brenner does to the patient what her father did to her. He generates a bait and switch where he (Brenner) is the authority of her life, free to replace her understanding of events with his own at his pleasing (Levenson, 2005; see also Chapter 2 for a more ongoing discussion of this).

To counter this dyadic meaning-making, Wilford Bion says, "[T]he capacity to forget, the ability to eschew desire and understanding, must be regarded as essential discipline for the psychoanalyst" (1988, p. 51). Lastly, Shoshana Felman, explicating her understanding of Lacan, says that we must remember that

> the psychoanalytical interpreter is not, himself, in possession the truth of his interpretation, does not possess, in other words, the unconscious discourse he delivers, because the truth of this unconscious discourse is ... radically dialogic (it can only come about, discursively, in analytic dialogue, it is neither in, or of, the analyst, nor in, or of, the patient). (1987, p. 125)

Returning to the semiotic: The role of co-genetic logic as a way of thinking triadically

One way to move beyond dyadic thinking that has been elaborated by cultural psychologists is through what is termed co-genetic logic. Developed initially as a behavioral logic by David P.G. Herbst (1976), cultural psychology (Valsiner, 1995, 2007; Tateo 2016) has elaborated Herbst's work, maintaining that when a distinction within a field is made it axiomatically and unconsciously creates an oppositional field of meaning. Thus, the distinction A (whatever this might be, but, for example, "real") evokes immediately an oppositional non-A field. This is represented as A <> non-A; or for our example Real <> non-Real. Taken together, A <> non-A comprises an irreducible whole of meaning. Within the triadic frame, this whole (A <> non-A) only exists in some respect to an interpretant. This means that as the object "real" is represented in some way to someone, part of what is represented, albeit in a dormant fashion, is its ("real") relationship to "non-real." It is the duality of the object (A <> non-A) that in part allows for elaboration.

From the semiotic perspective, when "real experience" is represented by one analyst to someone else (i.e., another analyst or a patient), not only is the concept of "real experience" as the analyst understands it signified but with that also comes the possibilities of "non-real experience." The patient or analyst as *interpretant* then can signify their understanding of the analyst's idea, not understand this idea or alternatively further elaborate and develop this idea. Notably, when dyadic and authoritarian systems prevail, claims of not understanding or the proposal of non-analyst-authorized ideas have been treated historically as resistance or defense. While this, indeed, might be the case, it also does not have to be. From a field perspective, how the patient or other interlocutor understands and interprets the "real experience"; how (the means by which) they formulate meaning (Stern, 2009) is more the focus than what specific meaning they formulate.

Notably, this does not mean that *anything goes*. As stated earlier, for Peirce signification occurs with respect to the "ground" or the "context" of signification. Similarly, while A ("real experience") may have clear boundaries and definition and non-A ("non-real experience") remains more open, the dynamic tension between the two fields constrains and limits meaning-making. Making meaning outside of this context and field could happen, but it would not likely be understood or, at the very least, require an explanation as to how the field has shifted.

Within this process, however, there is space for indeterminate meaning-making, such that non-real can mean and be constructed as many potential things, i.e., phantasy but also, dreams, imagination, possibly video games, books, and forth. As a whole, whereby non-A stands in relation and so is constrained by A, development is limited by parameters of the relationship between A and non-A. What differentiates co-genetic logic from dyadic system then is the following triadic relationship: There is (1) a primary distinction (A <> non-A); (2) of which one set is closed (A), and (3) one is open (non-A) (Tateo, 2016). This comprises an irreducible whole unit of analysis, which exists within a unique tension such that meanings can develop in the back and forth of dialogue.

Clinical application

Clinical work with patients to explore or deconstruct aspects of their narrative can also be reframed as elaborating aspects of this dynamic relationship. Take for example students whose identities are tied up in their academic performance. Their sense of self is contingent upon being a "good" student. In this context, "good" entails a rather closed meaning, determined by certain grades or a GPA. Elaborating upon "good" in therapy would not gain much traction – though one might still do so by say focusing upon the history of being a good student. Simultaneously, good creates a relationship with "non-good." Notably, while one aspect of this might be "bad," this move of contrast between good and bad is already a development of the field. Slowing down the process, to look at other possible meanings that might be entailed with "non-good" would allow for meaningful elaboration and possible development. Thus, "non-good" may also entail ideas of "working more than others" or "having to get help from tutors." Opening up these non-A fields for expression and elaboration allows for possible development of the field, i.e., the A <> non-A relationship.

Summary

In this chapter, we propose the primary importance of seeing that what is essential about our nature is not our individual "identity" but, rather, our disposition toward continuity and discontinuity. We have focused upon how our ongoing evolution in identities must acknowledge our forever state of incompletion, even as we ardently seek its opposite: completion. We consider how this process occurs through semiotics or the ways that we know the world through various types of representation. This required us to take a deep dive into the work of first Charles S. Peirce and then cultural psychology to see in detail how triadic systems can account for development and growth in ways that dyadic systems cannot. This enables us to appreciate that the tension between completion/incompletion is generative as a type of psychological aliveness especially when we can stand the tension around not knowing.

With this foundation in place, we are now in a position to look at how continuity/discontinuity and completion/incompletion demonstrates more specifically within the interpersonal realm. We are in a position to discuss how our agency as being fares in the relational mix with other beings. We can proceed to consider the consequences for our health, our vitality, when our search for continuity overlaps with another being's search for completion or when our search for discontinuity is thwarted by our interaction with an important other's anxious incompletion. When meaning-making loses this dialectical energy and "collapses" into what Sartre would call a thing "in-itself" rather than "for-itself" than we lose the healthy vitality of movement and become stuck in a less adaptive position.

Accordingly, in the next chapter, we will take up how we react to this interpersonal mix of completion and incompletion with particular existential positions, with particular organized ways of relating to others and otherness. To launch us toward this Anaïs Nin serves well. She says, "Life is a process of becoming, a combination of states we have to go through. Where people fail is that they wish to elect a state and remain in it. This is a kind of death" (1964, p. 1). We hear that Nin acknowledges the broad stroke of what life is; it is always a "becoming." Shakespeare, through *Richard II*, echoes this:

> Thus play I in one person many people,
> And none contented: Sometimes am I a king;
> Then treasons makes me wish myself a beggar,
> And so I am: Then crushing penury
> Persuades me I was better when a king;
> Then am I king'd again ...
> (1812/c. 1597, Act 5 Scene 5, lines 31–36, p. 108)

Notes

1 Webb and Sells note that "Thou are that" is from the Chandogya *Upanishad* (*tat tuam asi*) which stresses that the "real" self is both within and without, both transcendent and immanent, eternally unmoving and yet swifter in its motion than the wind and experienced only when we can calm our mind and lose its ego-self attachments (*Upanishads*, 1946, pp. 14–25, 64–78).
2 See Orzel (2015, July 8) for a layman's explanation of this.
3 Lacan is also said to have acknowledged Peirce's contribution to his thinking, but it is clearly less integrated into his work.

References

Beebe, B (2005). Mother-infant research informs mother-infant treatment. *Psychoanalytic Study of the Child*, *60* (1), 6–46. 10.1080/00797308.2005.11 800745.

Beebe, B & Lachmann, F (1998). Co-constructing inner and relational process: Self and mutual regulation in infant research and adult treatment. *Psychoanalytic Psychology*, *15* (4), 480–516. 10.1037/0736-9735.15.4.480.

Beebe, B & Lachmann, F (2003). The relational turn in psychoanalysis: A dyadic systems view from infant research. *Contemporary Psychoanalysis*, *39* (3), 379–409. 10.1080/00107530.2003.10747213.

Beebe, B & Lachmann, R (2014). The origins of attachment, *Infant research and adult treatment*. New York and London: Routledge.

Beebe, B, Lachmann, F, Markese, S, Buck, KA, Bahrick, LE, Chen, H (2012b). On the origins of disorganized attachment and internal working models: Paper II. An empirical microanalysis of 4-month Mother-Infant interaction. *Psychoanalytic Dialogues*, *22*, 352–374.

Bion, W (1988). *Attention and interpretation*. H. Karnac Books.

Borch-Jacobsen, M (1981). *Lacan: The absolute master*. Stanford University Press.

Brenner, C (1991). A psychoanalytic perspective on depression. *Journal of the American Psychoanalytic Association*, *39* (1), 25–43. 10.1177/00030651 9103900102

Erikson, E (1950). *Childhood and society*. W.W. Norton.

Felman, S (1985). *Jacques Lacan and the adventure of insight*. Harvard University Press.

Herbst, DPG (1976). Non-hierarchical forms of organization. Acta Sociologica, *19* (1), 65–75. 10.1177/000169937601900106.

Lacan, J (1982). A love letter. In J Mitchell & J Rose (Eds.), *Feminine sexuality: Jacques Lacan and the école freudienne* (pp. 149–161). W.W. Norton. (Original work published 1966).

Lacan, J (1977). *Ecrits: A selection* (A Sheridan, Trans.). W.W. Norton. (Original work published 1966).

Levenson, EA (1981). Facts or fantasies: On the nature of psychoanalytic data. *Contemporary Psychoanalysis*, *17*, 486–500.

Levenson, EA (2003). On seeing what is said: Visual Aids to the psychoanalytic process. *Contemporary Psychoanalysis*, *39* (2), 233–249. 10.1 080;00107530.2003.10745819.

Levenson, EA (2005). *The Ambiguity of Change*. Routledge Press. (Original work published 1983).

Mahler, M, Pine, F, & Bergman, A (2000). *The psychological birth of the human infant, Symbiosis and individuation*. Basic Books. (Original work published 1975).

Mitchell, S (1986). The wings of Icarus: Illusion and the problem of narcissism. *Contemporary Psychoanalysis*, *22* (1), 107–132. 10.1080/0010753 0.1986.10746118.

Nietzsche, F (1910). *The birth of tragedy or Hellenism and pessimism* (WA Haussman, Trans.). In O Levy (Ed.), *The complete works of Friedrich Nietzsche* (pp. 1–196). The Project Gutenberg EBook. (Original work published 1872).

Nin, A (1964). *D.H. Lawrence, an unprofessional study*. Swallow Press.

Orzel, C (2015, July 8). Six things everyone should know about physics. *Forbes Magazine.* https://www.forbes.com/sites/chadorzel/2015/07/08/six-things-know-quantum-physics/#59a7d8017d46.

Peirce, CP (1965). *The collected papers of Charles Sanders Peirce, V. 1–6* (C Hartshorne, C., & P Weiss, P, Eds.), *V. 7* (A Burks. Ed.). Harvard University Press.

Rosa, A (2007). Acts of Psyche: Actuations as synthesis of semiosis and action. In J Valsiner, J.& A Rosa (Eds.) *The Cambridge handbook of sociocultural psychology* (pp. 205–237). Cambridge, UK Cambridge University Press.

Rosenbaum, PJ & Webb, RE (2021). Appreciating Ogden's re-conceptualization of destruction but with a developmental arc: When is the big scary ape destructive? *Journal of Infant, Child, and Adolescent Psychotherapy.* Advance online publication. 10.1080/15289168.2021.1879711.

Sartre, J-P (1966). *Being and nothingness, a phenomenological essay on ontology* (HE Barnes, Trans.) Washington Square Press. (Original work published 1943).

Saussure, F. de (2006). *Writings in general linguistics* (S Bouquet & R Engler, Eds., C Sanders, M Pires, Trans.). Oxford University Press. (Original work published 2002).

Schore, JR & Schore, AN (2008). Modern attachment theory: The central role of affect regulation in development and treatment. *Clinical Social Work Journal, 36* (1), 9–20. DOI: 10.1007/s10615-007-0111-7.

Schneiderman, S (1990). Art as symptom: A psychoanalytic study of art. In PC Hogan & L Pandit (Eds.), *Criticism and Lacan on Language, Structure, and the Unconscious* (pp. 207–222). Univ. of Georgia Press.

Shakerspeare, W (2001). Richard II. In R Proudfoot, A Thompson, DS Kastan (Eds.), *The Arden Shakespeare, Complete Works* (rev.ed., p. 24). (Original work published c. 1595). Bloomsbury, IN.

Stern, DN (1983). *The Interpersonal World of the Infant: A View From Psychoanalysis and Developmental Psychology*. Basic Books.

Stern, DB (2009). *Partners in Thought: Working with Unformulated Experience, Dissociation and Enactment* (Psychoanalysis in a New Key Book Series). Routledge.

Tateo, L (2016). Toward a cogenetic cultural psychology. *Culture & Psychology, 22* (3), 433–447. 10.1177/1354067X16645297.

Upanishads (1946). *The Upanishads: Breath from the eternal mass*, S Prabhavananda & F Manchester (Translators). Mentor. (Original work composed 800-200 BCE).

Valsiner, J (1995). Processes of development, and search for their logic: An introduction to Herbst's co-genetic logic. In TA Kindermann, & J Valsiner (Eds.), *Development of person-context relations* (pp. 55–65). Lawrence Erlbaum Associates.

Valsiner, J (2007). *Culture in Minds and Societies: Foundations of Cultural Psychology*. Sage Publications.

Webb, RE & Sells, MA (1995). Lacan and Bion, Psychoanalysis and the mystical language of 'unsaying'. *Theory & Psychology*, *5*(2), 195–215. 10.1177/0959354395052002.

Whitehead, G (2010, May 24). A glossary of chickens. *The New Yorker*, *39*.

Winnicott, DW (1971). *Playing and reality*. Routledge Press.

Chapter 2

Introduction to Four Existential-Relational Positions

Having discussed our state of *being-ness* in the world and how we make meaning within our intra- and inter-personal relationships, we now turn our focus to the ways this unfolds. We propose that an ongoing challenge throughout life is navigating with a growing sense of agency and authority both our relationship of separation *from* others and our relationship of connection *to* others. We focus in this chapter on how this manifests developmentally in organizational states which we call "existential-relational positions."

While we view this process of individuation and self-authorization as ongoing and lifelong, it is important for our consideration of late adolescents and young adults, especially within the context of college and higher education. This age group is often in the throes of this process in ways that differ beyond simply its greater intensity from how it plays out later in life. Accordingly, we keep with the developmental and psychoanalytic literature which addresses how this process first occurs in early childhood, and also focus on how it emerges later in life, especially during adolescence and young adulthood.

What is existential about these positions?

Our thinking of these positions as existential reflects our efforts to integrate (and, at times, to interrogate) British Object Relations, existential philosophy and the ideas of Jacques Lacan. From our perspective, these positions relevantly pertain to how Donald Winnicott, a key clinical theorist in the early days of the object

DOI: 10.4324/9781003246558-3

relations school, says we use the *other* (the object) as an independent subject in order to become our own subject (Winnicott, 1969, 1971, 1975). Becoming a subject who can access agency within relationships is a key focus of ours. It also seems to us to be consistent with the existentialists' discussions about how we become a subject for-itself and not an object in-itself (Sartre, 1943/1966). Notably, we think the positions we describe encapsulate what Lacan (1968, 1978) has in mind when he elaborates about how agency and self-authorization emerge out of the pull and push we experience in seeking to be the completion of others while seeking the incompletion of ourselves. Since in a broad sense our focus is on depicting the sweep of *becoming*, we think it apt to call these organizations existential-relational positions.

Stable instability and linearity

In considering these existential-relational positions, we differentiate ourselves from emergent wholism where there is an assumption that development proceeds linearly with each stage building upon and subsuming the previous one in a kind of pyramidal way. We use the word "position," because, while these existential-relational organizations are linearly achieved, they do not subsume each other and thereby render the previous one in the succession no longer relevant (as the word "stage" can imply).

Instead, regardless of what position we achieve, we are always subject to movement between it and previous organizations. In this process, while achievement of a position might incline us to its more regular embodiment, such achievement is not stable. Movement between the positions reflects our varying ways of coping, consciously and unconsciously, with the demands of life. In certain contexts, and in the face of certain psychological stresses we can actively embrace or tumble into a particular position which might or might not be the one most recently, linearly achieved.

To a certain extent, then our "health" speaks to our ability to move flexibly between different ways of relating to self and others (Thompson, 1958) as we respond to life's challenges. However, our changing articulation of these existential-relational positions is not like marking up and then erasing a whiteboard so that we continually return to being a blank slate. The process of its articulation is more like layering of paper mache; our experiences always build, cover over and show through in the emerging iterations of our being.

These positions were originally named by clinical theorists of and influenced by the British object relations school (Grotstein, 2007; Klein, 1975a, 1975b; Ogden, 1986, 1989; Winnicott, 1975). Since this is so, we will rely on the foundational language of these theorists in describing these relational positions. However, we also will expand significantly on this language as we describe how these positions are achieved. In this regard, we will align ourselves with those who have applied considerable effort over the past forty years to reconcile cultural and interpersonal-relational sensibilities to the predominately internal, intra-psychic focus which was central to the original description and explanation of these positions. Pertinent to this John Padel, a psychoanalyst in training and practice during the early days of these positions' elaborations, tells an illustrative story. During a dinner, Winnicott told him: "I said to my analyst, I'm almost ready to write a book on the environment. She said to me, 'You write a book on the environment and I'll turn you into a frog!'" (Padel, 1989, p. 10). So, in the spirit of Winnicott, but perhaps even with more emphasis on the role of culture and interpersonal relationships we will risk becomes "frogs" in our elaborations of these developmental positions in the following sections.

Into the frog pond: The addition of cultural psychology

A dive into the frog pond of object relations entails recognition that developmental proceeds within the waters of culture. In other words, we recognize that ponds are situated within the ground of culture, as Peirce (1877) might say, and so inform where we are situated with respect to self and other. As we discussed in Chapter 1, this means that meaning-making must be understood within the context in which we swim. As an important aspect of this, we note here that semiotic or sign systems, our strokes for making meaning-making, are preadaptive. By this, we mean that semiotic systems help us prepare for the unknown waters by creating systems that are patterned and then habitual (Valsiner, 2007; Sullivan, 1953). It is through our ongoing conscious and unconscious semiotic mediation that we are able to construct ways of navigating our various human (and non-human) environments.

Thus, we might preemptively say that the existential-relational positions we introduce are reasonably thought of as mediating systems that help us to be in the world. That we move between and in and out of them speaks to the different ways we actively construct and negotiate our worlds. Hence, looking into the psychological processes that we and others see as underlying these meaning-making systems will allow us to better understand how these systems work (Rosenbaum & Webb, 2021; Webb & Rosenbaum, 2021a; Grotstein, 2007; Klein, 1975a, 1975b; Ogden, 1986, 1989; Winnicott, 1975). Along the way, we have to introduce a few ideas that help situate the cultural perspective. Not only do these provide context but we also think they may show how this perspective allows us to resolve some thorny conceptual issues.

Moving to developmental positions

The existential-relational positions that have been foundational to our ideas are as follows: "contiguous," "paranoid-schizoid," "depressive" and "transcendent."[1] These stages represent a way of thinking about how we are situated in the world with respect to:

1   Our sense of being a separate "I" in the world who recognizes the otherness of being-ness both in relation to others and to ourselves
2   Our experience of agency and embrace of self-authorization.

First position: Contiguous

The first position begins with birth and moves through the earliest months of development (i.e., 3–6 months). During the contiguous position, the child and the primary caregiver form an enmeshed unit. In our elaboration, we will refer to this caregiver as the M-other for reasons described in our introduction. In the contiguous position, the M-other is preoccupied with the needs of their baby and ideally attempts to meet them as seamlessly as possible. In this regard, a baby's cry signifies within the M-other the baby's needs and speaks to the level of closeness and attunement between them. The M-other's ability to interpret the baby's cries and other signs, of course, figures importantly in whether the M-other is able to offer the baby timely relief from hunger, being "wet," and so forth.

This is something which, of course, can never be done perfectly because dis-contiguity between the M-other and the child is something intrinsic to the relationship as soon as the child breathes air through their own lungs. Nonetheless, we reference contiguity in this position for two important reasons. First of all, as we noted earlier, it is something that the loving M-other seeks to maintain so that the baby's needs can be met in as optimally, non-stressful way as possible. Second, it is something which Lacan says the M-other seeks as a way to resolve their own incomplete, existential essence.

Lacan views the M-other's relationship to their child as being marked by a unique complication and challenge. M-other encourages the child toward the development and expression of their own identity, which involves separating and launching from their own personal orbit. Simultaneously, M-other or at least some of M-other is also unconsciously seeking to make the child their missing "phallus" (Lacan, 1966/1982). By this, Lacan means that some of M-other attempts to make the child the fulfillment of their existential incompletion, the signifier of what can never be signified. This can manifest in a variety of concrete ways that address M-other's ongoing efforts *at last* to encapsulate their own personal identity. In this way, the child can become an expression of M-other's own efforts to self-authorize with the result that the child can be under pressure to serve an impossible ontological function or accept roles that they are not developmentally prepared to meet because they cannot contest the demand and co-construct its meaning. Speaking to the challenges here, the psychoanalyst Jean Laplanche (1997) discusses the parental seduction of the child into their world as a way of recognizing the asymmetrical power dynamics at play and the need to tread lightly.

Phenomenologically speaking, the baby in the contiguous position is still insufficiently separate from the enmeshment with M-other to have a sense of otherness and, therefore, a sense of individual agency. While the baby may be demanding and expressing their needs, there is no deliberative agency at play. This also means that the baby's semiotic capacities are quite limited. The baby's capacity for meaning-making primarily reflects the baby's close attunement to M-other's interpretative capabilities and efforts. The following description brings together both the semiotic and relational processes to describe how this happens:

> The act of crying symbolically represents the infant's need in the mind of the interpreting mother. According to Sullivan, the crying behavior signifies "baby needs attention" in the mind of the mother. The infant's needs are communicated to the mother through the linguistic symbol (crying). In a symbolic sense, the child's needs exist in the mother and outside the child. From the Peircean perspective, the crying behavior of the infant is a symbol for: (1) infant's needs (object), and (2) an appeal for attention (meaning or interpretant in the mind of the mother. (Lincourt & Olczak, 1974, p. 35)

Throughout this process, mother works to create an average and expectable environment (Hartman, 1939/1958). However, as described in Chapter 1, babies are able to regulate their experience through their gaze, looking at and looking away from mother to moderate contact (Beebe, 2005; Beebe et al., 2012). Similarly, babies' cries are other rudimentary ways of navigating their overwhelming interpersonal environments.

We hasten to note here that although the contiguous position is rooted to our earliest experiences in the world, it is a position we can return to later in life, especially in times of heightened challenge to our usual sense of who we are. These times can fall upon us not only in times of extreme stress (trauma, see especially Chapter 6) but also in times of overwhelming elation. Of the latter, we reference the feeling of oneness that often accompanies spiritual ecstasy or the similar sense that especially accompanies the early throes of falling in love. The return to this "contiguous" feeling of oneness is something Shakespeare (1923) marvelously captures in Sonnet 39: "O how thy worth with manner may I sing,/When thou art all the better part of me?/What can mine own praise to mine own self bring,/And what is't but mine own, when I praise thee?" (p. 20).

Second position: Paranoid-schizoid position

In the second position, physical and psychological separateness begin to emerge for both the M-other and for the baby. This is considered to be an inevitable effect of aging and the socialization process and moves from about 9 months of age through early childhood (5–7 years). Notably, the distinct time of the paranoid-schizoid position is something continually debated and challenged. From our perspective of focusing on process and praxis, we are less concerned with *when* it occurs and more with *what* is occurring within the relational world of the infant (Stern, 1983).

During the move from the first position to the second position, the child's sense of self emerges from being one reflective of the M-other's pre-occupational image of them toward one's reflecting greater subjectivity and individuality. This occurs naturally as the child's needs become increasingly diverse and complex, representing their more developed physiological and psychological capacities and the correspondingly greater potential for dis-contiguity with M-other.

In parallel fashion, M-other's own needs, such as for adult companionship, work and even other children, also begin to emerge as an important factor as does, what Lacan (1993) calls, the "name of the father." With this phrase, Lacan is referencing the role of secondary caregivers, F-others, in supporting the aspect of M-other that knows the importance of pointing the baby's gaze in life away from being the phallus. This above mix of emerging complexities generates expected challenges in meeting the baby's needs in a seamless fashion, and as a result the baby (and mother) may experience doubt about and discomfort in how they are relating. We emphasize again, however, that a certain amount of disjunction or dis-contiguity in the relationship rhythm between M-other and child is inevitable, and, in fact, is important to the emergence of further development.

These early experiences of disjunction, far from being catastrophic, are the necessary requirements for the emergence of self-consciousness and agency, even if, at this point in our evolution of being-ness, they are rudimentary (Peirce, 1877; Sullivan, 1953). Disjunction, doubt, frustration and discomfort are all considered prompts which initiate processes that seek to overcome and/or make sense of these feelings in order to ensure continuous feelings of comfort and fulfillment. As we repeatedly note, it is important that the feelings of disjunction not be so great so as to overwhelm the child's capacities to regulate them more or less independently. When these feelings are too overwhelming, we as caregivers need to actively step into the child's orbit to help the child with the regulatposition from an "I" position (outsideion of their affective states so that the child can communicate their specific needs and have a better chance of having them met.

From a phenomenological perspective, we can thus hypothetically imagine that the baby's experience entails here a rudimentary sense of otherness and of agency. Their sense of otherness is restricted to that which is *me* and that which is *non-me*. In other words, the sense of otherness entails no developed or nuanced appreciation of the subjectivity of the other person. Others are experienced in a flat, a-contextual way.

Similarly, their sense of "me" is organized into their experiences in such a way as to help them make their interpersonal and intrapersonal worlds more stable, predictable and so safe. To do this, children begin to organize their experience of themselves into "good me" and "bad me" (Sullivan, 1953).

"Good me" speaks to experiences that lead to satisfaction and security from their primary caregivers, whereas "bad me" speaks to the experiences that cause their caregivers to become upset or angry and, consequently, to the child feeling insecure. "Not me" relegates to experiences that cannot be symbolized or abstracted. In efforts to further protect "good me," the child may project "bad me" out of them and into M-other (but also objects, such as loved toys). Hence, in preserving the "good" not only is M-other stable and predictable but the child is protected from retaliation that could result from Mother's anger at their (the child's) badness.[2] We describe in more detail these processes of "splitting" (i.e., good and bad) and "projection" (locating badness elsewhere) in Chapter 8 but note their essentialness to our being able to begin organizing and so both navigating and making meaning within our world.

Through this categorization and from the lens of co-genetic logic, we can also depict the relational field as me <> non-me. Note that our use here of non-me is different than the above description of the child's experience of themselves. Our use here of me/non-me speaks, instead, to the emergent semiotic field of self and other that comes about with the distinction of me. Thus, as children begin to experience a growing sense of themselves as a "me" they experience all that is outside of them and also the parts of themselves that are threatening as "non-me." As this is potentially overwhelming to them given their limited semiotic capacities, the non-me fields remain limited in their detail.

Agency, then, within this system is severely constrained. Since our experience is limited to the various types of "me" and only a simplistic view of the other (i.e., someone to be managed), the person functioning within the paranoid-schizoid position cannot recognize their agency in any meaningful way. This is because agency requires our understanding of context and difference in order for us to experience our capacity to choose. While the paranoid-schizoid position does offer some context, insofar as we can begin to organize experience into good and bad, without a fuller engagement with others we are not able to become subjects who know the limits of self and other.

In other words, the limited subjectivity of *me* and *not-me* within the paranoid-schizoid position mitigates against an appreciation of difference and otherness. As a result, true agentic expression is constrained, and the experience of choice is more akin to a feeling that what is chosen is ordained. It is simply the way it *should* be. Not surprisingly, then, when we interact with a "me" of the paranoid-schizoid position from an "I" position (outside of the paranoid-schizoid position), we may experience them as overly concrete, self-absorbed or as entitled.

In this respect, being within the paranoid-schizoid position almost always entails a defensive posturing (though see Chapter 8 for some important times it may not). When we are in the paranoid-schizoid position, both the difference of other people as well as our own felt difference (our badness) threatens our experiences of ourselves as "good-me." This challenges our sense of safety and security in the world and how we experience authority. If we view ourselves as bad or are in relationship with others who see us as "bad," we are at risk of being abandoned, attacked or generally hurt.

This dynamic informs in an important way how we then group together with others. We often seek the safety in affiliation with others, but since there is no competing difference that relativizes perspective, the only justifiable and mitigating authority come from "me" and persons "like me." Accordingly, this position may inform times we are devoted tribalists whose experience, if not explicit mantra involves splitting the world into those like us who "are the good" and those who are not like us "who are the bad." We will elaborate more on this aspect in Chapter 8 (Webb & Rosenbaum, 2021b).

Third position: Depressive position

It is in the third position, the depressive position, that the elaboration of "good me" and "bad me" begins to be explored in relationship to others in such a way that these others emerge as subjective beings. In contrast then to the *no sense* of otherness of the first position and the *me/not-me* relationship to otherness of the second position, in the third position *I* and *you* begin to emerge. In other words, others become persons with a context and contours that differ from our own in a way that is appreciated.

From the Lacanian perspective, we see this evolution of subjectivity as reflecting the ongoing role of the "name of the father" (Lacan, 1993). F-other supports the M-other in helping us as the child to see that our destiny is not found in attempts to authorize the completion of M-other. Instead, our destiny has to be found in pursuing our own incompletion, which is, of course, the essence of our own being-ness (Webb et al., 1996).

From vector of object-relations, we can see the developmental processes occurring at this phase what happens as the child moves from object relating to object usage. In Winnicott's famous paper, "The use of an object and relating through identification," he writes,

> A new feature thus arrives in the theory of object-relating [as it evolves into object-usage]. The subject says to the object: 'I destroyed you,' and the object is there to receive the communication. From now on the subject says: 'Hullo object!' 'I destroyed you.' 'I love you.' 'You have value for me because of your survival of my destruction of you.' 'While I am loving you I am all the time destroying you in (unconscious) *fantasy*.' (1969/ 1971, p. 90)

While this paragraph has been interrogated recently by Ogden (2016) and also by us (Rosenbaum & Webb, 2021), we want to note the semiotic capacity at play here. The child begins to develop a semiotic system by which they can say to the object (the other) that they love them, and they destroy them. In the words of Levenson (1981), they are "engaged in a circumscribed semiotic system" (p. 496). It is a system that becomes hierarchically organized; in other words, it develops.

Initially, the object receives the communication ("I destroyed you"); they thus serve as an interpretant of the subject and provide the burgeoning child the experience of being seen and witnessed. Afterward, the child can then say "hello" to the object and thereby brings them into recognition as well. They then say, "I destroyed you. I love you." The past tense of destruction speaks to one set of experiences, and the present tense of "I love you" speaks to another. The object is thus both destroyed and loved. The object, the person who is other, is able to embody both our aggression/assertion and our love. The object's survival of our aggression allows for the appreciation of this other's subjective and independent state of being, and in this regard this other's survival provides its semiotic value as a tool to help the child navigate the world. The object's survival emerges as a higher-level symbol, hierarchically organizing the child's experience such that it is okay to destroy and to love since they know that the object will survive. Love and destruction are brought under semiotic control and internalized, albeit for Winnicott in fantasy.

Looking more closely at this process, the crucial aspect of this communication is the way that the object becomes internalized by surviving the destruction. Survival here is equated as not retaliating against the child's destructive actions. For Winnicott (1969/1971) and Ogden (2016), the child destroys because they are upset at the parent's failure (however inevitable and necessary) to meet their needs. In Winnicott's words, "destruction turn[s] up" (p. 91).

We think, however, that we can reframe this failure of contiguity not only as expected but also as a necessary part of the developmental process that fosters the child's increasing socialization. Thus, destruction occurs not only out of anger but also as part of the exploration of the non-A fields, regardless of what those fields might be. Exploration of non-A fields, in other words, is a required part of our emergence as a being, because *becoming* requires delimitation; it requires experiencing other ways of being. As the parent socializes certain aspects of the child, they axiomatically introduce other fields for discovery. In their less socialized and so more open and wonderous way, the child expands the non-A field in such a way that the parent can feel challenged and even destroyed.

For example, as the parent says to the child that "they love them" they are also introducing the non-"they love them" field. Children unconsciously and unreflectively may explore this non-field by articulating the ways that the parent, indeed, does not love them. For instance, consider the three-year-old, who in reeling from not getting something they want, yells "I hate you"; "I don't want to see you"; "You're not nice to me. How are we to understand this? Is this a child intentionally trying to destroy the object?" From a cultural perspective, it would not make sense to attribute the child with self-reflective agency here but instead to think about them as exploring the limits of the non-loving field. They are, in other words, utilizing agency to explore potentiality and enable the emergence of other ways of being.

It is through the parents' (and child's) repetition and ongoing survival (without retaliation) that the child comes to see the parameters of that field (the ground as it were). Notably, survival does not mean that there is no discomfort or rupture. A parent whose told by the child that "I hate you" may have a strong emotional reaction which gets communicated to the child. This creates the feelings of discomfort that are essential for prompting new exploration and growth. In turn, this enables further distinctions in development. The distinction of "I love you"/"I destroy you" speaks to ways of being which entails both loving and destroying. Semiotically, the child is beginning to be able to use other people as objects within their own world while recognizing the object's subjectivity.

Within the object-relations theory, the feelings of discomfort noted earlier are specifically connected to feelings of guilt and shame at having hurt a loved object. The experience of these feelings and the need to navigate the difficulties that experiencing them creates is what prompts the movement from the second to the third positions. We begin to learn that the distinctions of "good" and "bad" that reside within us also reside within others. With this we, then, come to see that those who are not-me are other "I's" ("you's"), and we also begin to understand that how they exist in the world is appreciably more complicated than any simple categorization as either good or bad provides. In grappling with this, the child, lastly, begins to deal with growing awareness of incompletion and the bounded limits of being-ness both for themselves and for others. Awareness of their agency in the dynamic of this emerges.

The fostering of this growing awareness of our incomplete essence as beings and of the inherent complexity of good and bad launches us into the fourth existential-relational position.

Fourth position: Transcendence

So far, we have traced a developmental progression that occurs in relationship to primary and secondary caregivers whose otherness becomes both increasingly apparent and tolerable/embraceable. We move from having no sense of otherness in the contiguous position to a more developed sense of I and you in the depressive position. Similarly, our capacity for agency and self-authorization also develops from no sense of agency toward eventually a relativized sense of agency.

With our step into the transcendent position, we come not only to tolerate difference but to enjoy and seek it out. However, our capacity to authorize ourselves as creative and worthy meaning-making agents (as we do when we are within the transcendent position) hinges upon a final important step. Our F-other and the M-other must invite us to recognize and accept both the relativity and the limitation of their authority and knowledge as beings in the world. In other words, they must invite us to embrace a wondering about life that acknowledges that life extends both to different ponds and even to life outside of ponds.

The role of our key caregivers at this point, then, is to lead the child out of being the completion of another's being and to recognize ultimately the constructive nature of meaning that occurs within culture and language. Staying within the parlance of Lacan, we say that the F-other introduces the child to the "Law," a process accomplished when the "father (sic) does not make the child the object of his desire and is not the desire of the child [but understands and communicates that] he does not have the phallus as the satisfaction of desires but as a symbol" (Webb et al., 1996, p. 9). The "law", in other words, is that we all must recognize that we are, whether labeled a "frog" or "fish," dwellers within a pond. We are all situated *somewhere*. This being so, we can imagine that in other breathing spaces, whether in water or not, we can name ourselves and others differently.

The process of coming to recognize the constructive reality of identity and culture comes with the potential for joy and dread. The joy lives in the liberation felt in being able to see the space for our own agency in defining who we are. In our embrace of that joy, we self-authorize. A dread, however, can also be felt. The transcendent position requires that we embrace our existential responsibility to accept that there is no specific identity or state of being that is essentially our own and simply awaiting our discovery. Our essence, instead, is always incompletion seeking completion, and we, each of us, are responsible for the embrace of this dynamic which makes us not only always "other" to others but "other to ourselves."

Thus, to move into the transcendent position, parents and others who serve in the F-other role must be willing to be de-authorized as expert in knowing the destiny of their child's life. This can be painful for the parent who perhaps has enjoyed basking in the idealization of their child. Yet, it is what we must do as parents even while working to avoid granting too much agency and authority to children who are experimenting with different iterations of themselves and doing so still with an active illusion that there is an essential self within themself for which, in the absence of parental authorization, there is other truth-knowing authority.

Complexities in transitioning between positions

The developmental progression from one position to another is rarely smooth and without issue. As alluded to earlier, during development (especially in its earliest periods) we hope for average and expectable and good enough conditions. However, challenges erupt somewhere along the developmental continuum for everyone in life's negotiation. We might say that we fall "ill" when we hit a bump in the road that puts us out of the trek forward. In other words, we become compromised psychologically when we get so overwhelmed that we fall into a stagnating stasis in our sense of being-ness; we fall into a state where our incomplete essence is stymied, and we, therefore, stop feeling the aliveness that marks our evolving iterations of personhood.

This can happen for reasons that centrally reflect the particulars of a specific child-parent relationship but can also more immediately reflect the serendipity of contextual factors that weigh in beyond the control of this dyad. For example, those who suffer from trauma, poverty, marginalized social identity and so forth often face considerably greater risk and substantial difficulties in both achieving the paranoid-schizoid position and being able to move toward the depressive one. While much of the object-relations and attachment literature recognizes and even comes out of situations where care struggles to be good enough (i.e., Bowlby (1988) working with orphans post-World War II or Beebe's (2005) work, with mother's following 9/11), a normative tilt toward what is White, European, heteronormative, neurotypical and affluent still predominates. Accordingly, our forays into the various developmental challenges, impasses, and stagnations require recognition that systemic factors (biological, social and cultural) play significantly in how smoothly development can proceed. In other words, once we embrace being a frog of one particular kind or another, we also realize that the ponds into which we are born and within which we swim can be very different.

While notably, many of our ensuing chapters deal precisely with the ways that problems ensue in acquisitions of the latter three positions, but especially the paranoid-schizoid and depressive positions, it is important to say a few words here about what we see broadly as occurring. In considering our emergence from dependent toward greater amounts of independence we are susceptible to relational pulls by which our primary caregivers for whatever reason are challenged to see our subjectivity and meet our needs in as a smooth way as possible. This creates various potentials for developmental stagnations and impasses which occur when our passage through positions is thwarted.

Challenges in going from contiguous to paranoid-schizoid

The movement from the contiguous to the paranoid-schizoid position can be challenging for numerous reasons. For instance, the movement from the contiguous to paranoid-schizoid can be complicated when the baby is not able to internalize good enough object experiences. This sometimes results when the parent has been traumatized and so becomes impatiently angry at the child because their basic needs seem to exceed what the parent sees as typical. In short, there are times when the parents, because of their own unique histories, respond to the child's needs with a feeling that is disproportionate to the frustration that is usually inherent to providing good care.

Alternatively, parents, because of the shadow of their own pre-parenting history, may dissociate when interacting with the baby and, therein, confuse the baby with experiences that are either over- or under-stimulating. In these interactions, the child cannot adequately encode their experiences into a sense of "good-me" and thereby draw out predictable responses from the parent. Consequently, their movement into the paranoid-schizoid position is challenged by intense feelings of fear or confusion about the *other*. While most children achieve, even if only partially, some paranoid-schizoid functioning and, thereby, are able to organize the world into stable and predictable good and bad terms, in these cases the potential for chaotic psychological disorganization is a very real and serious possibility. In this case, we can say that the field of A <> non-A is so constrained that conditions are not truly safe enough for A to be meaningful.

Challenges in going from paranoid-schizoid to depressive

Similar constraints exist within the paranoid-schizoid position as the child learns to navigate the increasing complexities of self and other. Here, the child has to be able, in the parlance of Winnicott (1971), to destroy the object in order to find the object. This destruction, which is a blend of real action and phantasy, has to be held appropriately within the grounds of the situation. If it is lost because the M-other cannot bear being "destroyed," the semiotic field becomes overly constrained and a developmental impasse is at hand.

Destruction as a prerequisite for further development also can be considered usefully here from the perspective of Lacan. He speaks of this situation as being one where the child cannot emerge into their own incomplete being if they feel constrained to being the completion of M-other (Lacan, 1966/1982). Accordingly, as the child begins to assert themselves through needs which challenge the M-other's intolerance of their own incompleteness, the Mother's capacities to love even while the child may be destructive is compromised. The phrase, toddler terrorist, comes here to mind. Surviving this period entails allowing for A to be destroyed by the child and holding onto the potential for other meanings (non-A). This helps the M-other with not retaliating against the child and allows them perspective to see the child as attempting to differentiate themselves and their being. If M-other must cling too anxiously onto sustaining A, an impasse is at hand.

Challenges in going from depressive to transcendent

Things get further complicated because it is just not M-other who is a parental player. There is also F-other. The F-other must be able to support the side of M-other that knows that the child cannot be the phallus of completion. The F-other must aid in the caregiving to insist that the child relinquish this inclination to try and complete M-other. However, this F-other function has its own complexity. The F-other must not point the child to a destiny that is outside of being M-other's missing "phallus" only then to insist, in a kind of bait and switch maneuver, that child admires F-other's phallus. Within the depressive position, the F-other has to relinquish the hegemony over naming to allow for depressive mourning and ultimately the child's greater exploration of non-A. A failure at doing this can prompt a turn of the child toward manic denial of limitation or present other significant difficulties with integrating the loss that is intrinsic to F-other process, all of which can obstruct the move toward the transcendence position where self-authorization is truly achieved.

The disappointments of life

A key feature, then, of the challenges embedded in all the transitions from one position to another is dealing with the disappointments and losses of life. In this regard, it is often during the latter years of childhood (10–13) that children begin to grasp and appreciate that they cannot be good at all things. Hence, they begin to reckon with and embrace incompletion and glimpse life's tragic nature (Mitchell, 1994). This again is a mixed bag which generates depressive feelings and a need to mourn losses but also avenues of new exploration. Not being good at all things means being good at some things. It is this balance that gives the depressive position its flair and nurtures empathy and understanding toward self and other.

For example, a problem we've long noted in working with perceptive and bright college aged students is the burgeoning professionalism of these early years. Too many students belatedly seem to face developmental concerns that have been superseded by the need, even at this early age, to build an impressive academic resumé. This, of course, in some measured way can be an adaptive response on the parent's part to the larger pressures of our modern world. However, it may also reflect the parent's own struggle with integrating depressive position disappointment and loss which they deal with by focusing in a manic way on the "winning" and "excellence" of the extension of their being which they find located in their child.

Regardless of the basis for this focus, there seems to us to be an ongoing creeping of it into earlier and earlier school grades. This poses a significant danger to the psyches of children and early adolescents who are detoured away from coming to terms with finding their own desires and paths. By their college days they are living a life of empty despair (they don't feel their aliveness from within themselves), and they sometimes then, in the best scenario, crumble into a "better late than never identity crisis" wherein they feel compelled to seek, however vaguely, resonance with life that feels more centrally located from within their own being.

Hence, when we as parents or even when the institutions we are members of fail to embrace and integrate our own depressive anxiety, we are susceptible to a paranoid-schizoid stance where we generate hyper-regulated fields of meaning that are overly constricted and narrow. In the example above, when we cannot tolerate the disappointment and anxieties that our children's' educational journeys entail, we can fall prey to hyper-regulating the field of potential meanings (A) and find ourselves adamantly insistent upon admission into certain schools or involvement only in a particular set of extracurriculars. Friendships or hobbies for our children which don't directly serve the achievement goal upon which we have fixated meaning are actively discouraged. This, of course, does not necessarily mean that the child does not engage in them, but they may do so in secret or even at the expense of their academics.

Summary

In this chapter, we articulated four existential-relational positions which we achieve linearly (but not in an emergent wholistic way) as we incorporate into our life individuation in relation to otherness, agency and self-authorization, and the incompletion of being-ness. The path this development takes allows for increasing capacity to sustain relatedness in open and curious ways, though, as we note, it can be threatened by stagnation at numerous points in time. These existential-relational positions and the ongoing psychological processes that inspired them inform not only our sense of development but, most importantly, also how we work clinically with patients. Accordingly, we turn to these implications in the next chapter before describing specific issues that emerge along the path.

Notes

1 See our introduction for a discussion of the historical naming of these positions and our slight shift in terminology.
2 We recognize the somewhat quick synthesis here of Sullivan's descriptive states of "good me," "bad me and "not-me" and Klein's processes of projection and splitting. To us, this synthesis makes sense and is consistent with the relational trend of integrating interpersonal and object relations (see, for instance, Mitchell, 1994). Understandably, some may want us to slow this down and further discuss each metatheory and how they are situated, which we do somewhat more in Chapter 6 where we consider trauma and Chapter 7 where we discuss in greater detail projection and splitting.

References

Beebe, B (2005). Mother-infant research informs mother-infant treatment. *Psychoanalytic Study of the Child*, *60* (1), 6–46. 10.1080/00797308.2005.11 800745

Beebe, B, Lachmann, F, Markese, S, Buck, KA, Bahrick, LE, Chen, H (2012). On the origins of disorganized attachment and internal working models: Paper II. An empirical microanalysis of 4-month Mother-Infant interaction. *Psychoanalytic Dialogues*, 22, 352–374.

Bowlby, J (1988). *A secure base*. New York, Routledge Classics.

Hartmann, H (1958). *Ego psychology and the problem of adaptation* (D Rapaport, Trans.). International Universities Press. (Original work pub-lished 1939)

Grotstein, JS (2007). The concept of the "transcendent position." In J Grotstein (Ed.), *A beam of intense darkness, Wilfred Bion's legacy to psychoanalysis* (pp. 121–134). Karnac Press. 10.4324/9780429471209-1

Klein, M (1975a). *The collected works of Melanie Klein, Volume I, love, guilt and reparation and other works 1921–1945*. The Free Press.

Klein, M (1975b). *The collected works of Melanie Klein, Volume III, envy, gratitude and other works 1946–1963*. The Free Press.

Lacan, J (1968). *Speech and language in psychoanalysi*s (A Wilden, Trans.). Johns Hopkins University Press. (Original work published 1956).

Lacan, J (1978). *The four fundamental concepts of psychoanalysis* (J Miller, Ed. & A Sheridan, Trans.). Norton. (Original work published 1956).

Lacan, J (1982). The meaning of the phallus. In J.Mitchell & J Rose (Eds.), *Feminine sexuality, Jacques Lacan and the école Freudienne* (pp. 74–85). Norton. (Original work published 1966).

Lacan, J (1993). *The psychoses, The seminar of Jacques Lacan. Book III 1955–1956* (J-A Miller, Ed. & R Grigg, Trans.). Routledge.

Laplanche, J (1997). The theory of seduction and the problem of the other. *International Journal of Psychoanalysis*, *78* (4), 653–666.

Levenson, EA (1981). Facts or fantasies: On the nature of psychoanalytic data. *Contemporary Psychoanalysis*, *17*, 486–500.

Lincourt, JM & Olczak, PV (1974). C.S. Peirce and H.S. Sullivan on the human self. *Psychiatry*, *37* (1), 78–84. 10.1080/00332747.1974.11023789

Mitchell, SA (1994). *Hope and dread in psychoanalysis*. Basic Books.

Ogden, TH (1986). *The matrix of the mind, Object relations and the psychoanalytic dialogue*. Jason Aronson Inc.

Ogden, TH (1989). *The Primitive edge of experience*. Jason Aronson Inc.

Ogden, T (2016). Destruction reconceived: On Winnicott's 'The use of an object and relating through identifications'. *International Journal of Psychoanalysis*, *97* (5), 1243–1262. 10.1111/1468-5922.5922.12341

Padel, J (1989, March 10). *The psychoanalytical theories of Melanie Klein and Donald Winnicott and their interaction in the British Society of Psychoanalysis* [Paper presentation]. Philadelphia Society for Psychoanalytic Psychology, Spring Meeting.

Peirce, CP (1877). The fixation of belief. *Popular Science Monthly*, *12*, 1–15.

Peirce, CP (1965). *The collected papers of Charles Sanders Peirce, V. 1–6* (C Hartshorne, C., & P Weiss, P., Eds.), *V. 7* (A Burks. Ed.). Harvard University Press.

Rosenbaum, PJ & Webb, RE (2021). Appreciating Ogden's re-conceptualization of destruction but with a developmental arc: When is the big scary ape destructive? *Journal of Infant, Child, and Adolescent Psychotherapy*. Advance online publication. 10.1080/15289168.2021.1879711

Stern, DN (1983). *The Interpersonal World of the Infant: A View From Psychoanalysis and Developmental Psychology*. Basic Books.

Sartre, J-P (1966). *Being and nothingness, a phenomenological essay on ontology* (HE Barnes, Trans.) Washington Square Press. (Original work published 1943).

Shakespeare, W (1923). Sonnet 39. In WL Cross & T Brooke (Eds.), The Yale Shakespeare, (p. 20). (Original work published 1609). New Haven, CT: Yale Publications.

Sullivan, HSS (1953). *The interpersonal theory of psychiatry*. New York: W.W. Norton Publications.

Thompson, M (1958). *The death of desire: A study in psychopathology*. New York University Press.

Valsiner, J (2007). *Culture in Minds and Societies: Foundations of Cultural Psychology*. Sage Publications.

Webb, RE, Bushnell, DF, & Widseth, JC (1996). The birth and death of desire: the Significance of Lacan's "Name of the Father" in work with the sexually abused. *Clinical Studies: International Journal of Psychoanalysis, 2* (2), 1–22.

Webb, RE & Rosenbaum, P (2021a). Embracing diversity: The complexities of reckoning and accepting otherness. *Integrative Psychological and Behavioral Science, 50* (1), 30–46. DOI: 10.1007/s12124-020-09582-9.

Webb, RE & Rosenbaum, PJ (2021b). Tribalism: Where George Orwell leads us and where an understanding of existential-relational positions extends us. *The ory & Psychology*. Advance online publication. 10.1177/0959354321998776

Winnicott, D (1969). The use of an object and relating through identifications. *International Journal of Psychoanalysis, 50*, 711–716.

Winnicott, DW (1971). *Playing and reality*. Routledge Press.

Winnicott, DW (1975). *Through pediatrics to psycho-analysis*. Basic Books.

Chapter 3

Clinical Implications and Posture

Guiding therapeutic values and orientations

Consideration of our existential-relational situated-ness has important implications that inform our conceptualization, understanding and clinical interventions with student-patients throughout the ensuing chapters. How and where we see someone (not to mention ourselves) along a developmental continuum that relates to our embrace of otherness, individuation, agency and self-authorization is key to our capacity for making meaning and tolerating the ambiguity that shapes the therapeutic process. It is central to the questions we ask and the interpretations we offer. Similarly, it is helpful to us in guiding our relational engagement with patients since we often only can come to understand where someone is with respect to these questions after periods of engagement, exploration, conflict and so forth.

Accordingly, in this chapter, we outline with broad strokes some of the ways existential-relational positions figure in our clinical considerations, including some of the ways we sustain and engage in relationships differently, depending upon how and when our patients are situated in these positions. As stated in the introduction, our theory, in most respects, emerges from our clinical experiences of working in college counseling, private psychotherapy and psychoanalysis. Our path in exploring the clinical theories of object-relations, Lacan and interpersonal psychoanalysis has led also to theoretical abstraction in existentialism, phenomenology and semiotic mediation. We think the mix of all of this has helped us

DOI: 10.4324/9781003246558-4

greatly in our struggle to make sense of and understand our patients and ourselves. So, while at times we may take a more philosophically minded approach, we do so, because we have found it useful for centering ourselves as we work to initiate and sustain meaningful therapeutic relationships, often with individuals who have suffered tremendous trauma in their lives.

We think the need for flexible but sophisticated and nuanced theory to help us understand and sustain *ourselves* in often-challenging therapeutic relationships has motivated our clinical and theoretical exposition. We, of course, do not think ourselves to be uncommon in this regard. Clinicians have to construct and re-construct theory anew with each patient in order for it to be personally and clinically meaningful. Any overtly top-down application of theory onto a relationship rather than a bottom-up building of theory runs the real risk of alienation, forced compliance and possible harmful reenactment.

Hence, while we offer a theory of development about how we move through different positions in our efforts to relate to ourselves and others, we do not view this as something to be applied like a template. We offer our developmental model, instead, with the hope that it serves as a "stir" rather than an "instruction" about how within the therapeutic relationship we consider agency, authorization, otherness and individuation. Moreover, we see the relationship to the patient as always in the foreground. The emphasis is on the meaning that we and patients, as the dyad, construct with each other, and the effort is to create and hold space which can be used increasingly by patients for spontaneous and authentic expression of their experience in the world.

While our perspective values transference and countertransference dynamics, there is less emphasis on clearing up distorted relationships and more of an investment in determining why and how a patient and analyst are experiencing each other in particular ways. Similarly, unconscious processes and motivations matter tremendously, but rather than seeing these as teleological expressions of drives or certain developmental conflicts, our effort is to understand how patterned ways of relating to self and other have emerged or stalled in real relationships.

Our model of existential-relational development and semiotic mediation allows for highlighting a few aspects of clinical theory and technique. These are as follows:

1   In meeting with patients, we think about where they are currently situated with respect to how they relate to self and other, agency and authorization. Our developmental model serves a reference that we hold, not always in a conscious and disciplined way, but as a resource for helping us to find a foothold in our work. In this, it helps us to ask specific questions about ourselves and our patient that can be of use in framing our work. This is especially helpful when we are feeling lost or uncertain.

2   Our questions often reflect a broad feeling of where our patients are located with respect to their relating to self-object-other (Marková, 2003a, 2003b). This is akin to a form of triangulation similar to that of global positioning satellites (GPS) involving semiotic mediation and Peirce's ideas of semiosis (1965). For example, where we implicitly and explicitly see ourselves and our patient situated developmentally and relationally influences whether we choose to ask questions that are more object oriented than oriented toward the self.

3   In agreement with the work of Donnel Stern (2006, 2009, 2015), from our perspective, it is crucial that there is "movement" within the field. Movement is a broad term, but within our specific semiotic perspective it means an elaboration of some form of A or non-A. Elaboration here can take two forms. It can be toward more articulation, such that someone comes in with a story where they had a sense of what they are feeling and so work to amplify it. It can also mean a deconstruction of a tightly held narrative.

4   We view the embodied and situated being of therapist and patient as crucial to generating movement within the field. What each party brings into it is what is available for semiosis, including what they are conscious and unconscious of. Accordingly, utilizing our experience within the therapy space can be an important source of not only information but also signification. If we can, for instance, not only acknowledge feeling bored but be curious about that feeling and associate to it within the consulting room, we are convinced that this impacts the ongoing relatedness between patient and therapist in

truly significant ways. In this, we value the capacity of the therapist to help regulate (Schore & Schore, 2008) our patient's emotional and relational experience. Elaboration of the field of relatedness hopefully will allow for more freedom and a greater range of expression on the part of the patient and therapist.

5   Finally, we note the possibility for tremendous flexibility and creativity within the field. Patients and therapists alike can and do move between positions within the same session and make multiple meanings of the same event.

Some thoughts about the different positions

In thinking about how patients relate to us, as we noted earlier, we find it useful to wonder where they are positioned developmentally. How they engage us and our otherness to them impacts the field and informs how we might respond to them to encourage movement either between positions or within positions. The below summary is not meant to be comprehensive but rather a brief sketch of questions and ideas that have come into words for us as we position ourselves with patients from the perspectives we enumerate above. We are always in the process of reviving and revising this. We especially focus on how our work shapes itself when we experience ourselves as interacting with patients who are in the first two existential-relational positions, the contiguous and paranoid-schizoid. It is in these positions where we think we as therapist are most challenged to be creative in how we register our understanding and then respond to our patients. This is not to say that work with patients in the third and fourth positions, the depressive and transcendent, is not challenging. However, since the work from within these positions is more firmly based in the "world of words," more conventional perspective about what we do as therapists applies.

Sitting with patients when they are in the contiguous position

When working with patients in the contiguous position we make a distinction between whether they are there as a result of a "collapse" or because of lack of care. If it is the former, it is likely due to an overwhelming experience such as discrete trauma, intense affect

(shame/fear) or because they are in the throes of an early loving relationship or impassioned immersion in a group ideology. In the case
of lack of care, early life experiences have resulted in insufficient
foundation for making other developmental positioning possible.

When there has been a collapse

If we believe that the patients' contiguous experiencing is a result of
"collapse," we may respond in a bracing and structuring way with the
intention of slowly inviting them to envision positioning and perspective that we believe they either have achieved previously or are
yet capable of achieving. At times, however, this may entail our
concrete endorsement of their need to accomplish certain tasks, such
as self-care, hygiene or schoolwork. The thinking here reflects the
understanding that the collapse is in response to life events and while
processing it is, of course, important, it may take a back seat to more
pressing "real life" concerns. Indeed, we consider the times when we
sometimes say to patients to focus on their work or get four hours of
sleep as one of the distinguishing factors between practicing in a
college counseling center and other settings.

Still, other times, the student's collapse might be more profound
and manifest in ways that go sufficiently beyond a stymied ability to
do academic work that even basic self-care is in jeopardy. In these
circumstances, meeting the student on the "turf" onto which they
have landed can be of paramount importance.

For example, we recall an instance toward the end of the fall semester when a student near completion of his degree was suddenly
frozen in his capacity to do academic work. His suitemates out of
concern called CAPS and a therapist went to the dorms to meet the
student there. The student was sitting on the floor with the window
open and cold wind bristling about. The therapist joined the student
on the floor to enter into *the diffusion* and to accept the *space* that the
student had chosen for talking.

Working slowly, the therapist balanced the need to hear what was
happening with the fragility and tenderness of the student. So the
therapist, after a good while on the floor, said, "I want to know more
about your situation, but I'm cold and fear that I won't be able to
listen carefully enough if I don't get myself warm. May I close the

window?" Here, of course, we are inviting the student to accept that our and the student's self-care can be "other" to the story that is being told. In other words, self-care can be valued even while we value (immerse ourselves in) the story. And from this point, we proceed step by step until *maybe* we can get the student to connect to "home" or go to a hospital or some other safe place because it now feels sensible to them within the story they have shared in an inter-personal way. It feels "sensible" because we have worked as therapist to contextualize how doing this situates itself meaningfully within the diffusion that prevails.

These concrete interventions, far from the therapist "acting out" a desire to be heroic, reflect an understanding of the patient's existential-relational positioning. At times, it is enough to remain within the more traditional role of talking things through such that the patient can feel motivated themselves to "get back up and off the floor." However, often times, especially when there has been trauma, what is emergently needed is intervention wherein we *not only* tune ourselves to where the patient is but, in the service of preventing loss of life or deep descent into psychosis, we embody the agency and authority that was once the patient's but now in their diffusion cannot hold onto.

When there is a lack of care

When patients present themselves in the contiguous fashion not out of a collapse that we can determine but more from their own early attachment trauma, we often experience them in more diffuse and dissociated ways. As a result of the accompanying dysregulation, especially early on in treatment, we may not experience ourselves as having a lot of room for our own thinking, feeling and associative processes. The effects of these attachment traumas are topics we take up throughout this book (see especially Chapters 5 and 6) since the lack of stable base is reflected in any number of developmental im-passes that both speak to and generate trauma.

From our clinical perspective, what we want to highlight here are some of the clinical implications for working with patients in this position. Here, we feel that we need to hold in mind that the ex-pression of our own subjectivity and agency, if not carefully regulated by us, can easily overwhelm the patient and sustain how foreclosed they are from feeling that *within otherness* there is the possibility of creating meaningful connection. For instance, being with these patients can entail sitting through long periods of silence with what can feel like an absence of language and symbolization. *Offering* our own subjectivity as a way of musing about and entering into this silence is contribution we should consider. On the other hand, *filling* in this silent gap with the "authority" of our privileged role is another, and one we should consider only when dire circumstances of safety dictate it. The difference between "offering" and "filling," even if subtle, is critically important.

Indeed, sometimes, the way these patients present frustrates therapists in what seems like their resistance to doing the therapeutic work. Their vulnerability can easily be expressed in ways that feel like hostility to relating and relationship. Sustaining a relationship is thus the primary challenge and requires a therapist to be flexible in working to find and draw out the patient. As these patients often have true difficulties using language to depict their internal experiences, we are sometimes called to put words and language to them. This is the "offering" we noted earlier, and it is done tentatively and hesitantly on the part of the therapist who's sensitive to the ways that this may repeat or enact earlier relational trauma where the patients' forays into naming themselves were prohibited or squashed (the "filling" of above). Notably though, when done with real love, care, and concern this offered language can help scaffold patients' attempts to articulate their own inner experience and provide meaningful experiences of being seen and known in ways that have been otherwise lacking.

There are other notable times when patients often present in the contiguous position as well. This includes periods of rapturous love where they feel someone else has completed them. We might also think of patients who are described as "manic" as also residing in a defensive fashion within this position. They feel entirely as if some activity or pursuit will define them completely and fully. Indeed, one need not necessarily be manic to know the feeling of being completely and totally "understood" or "gotten." Notably though, a key semiotic distinction between when this reflects more paranoid-schizoid positioning versus autistic-contiguous is in the ability to use language to express what is being experienced.

Approach and questions in the contiguous position

Our approach with the contiguous position and the type of questions we ask reflect the following perspectives and effort:

1   We seek to "join" the patient in hearing the story that is fundamental to their current state of dissolution of their sense of being a separate person with a feeling of agency and authority. Thus, we recognize that they do not feel authentic (and likely have not been enabled to). Accordingly, we work to enter into the story with the patient so that we can begin to be a placeholder for the patient's suspension of their broader agency and authority for regulating their being-ness in wider life. In short, we must "join" before we can discuss any return to separation and embrace of "difference."

2   Our questions then are about the nature of their experience. They may be simple reflective questions, such a "tell me more about that" that to amplify a certain affect or important word or affect. Thus, our inquiry focuses mostly on their affective state with an effort to help formulate this for both them and for us. What is of importance at this phase is a sense of unobtrusiveness (Grossmark, 2018). We aim to be good "house guests" who do not make messes but rather walk softly and carefully. We reflect our care and concern not only in what we say, but how we say it, paying particular attention to tone, posture, sensitivity to eye contact, and so forth. Moreover, we may use our own experience with them in ways to help them put language to feelings and affect states (Quillman, 2012). In this, we understand that we are implicitly and explicitly helping patients regulate their experience and develop a sense of the shape and nuance of their own interiority.

3   In certain circumstances, we recognize that patients lack the words to populate their experience. Then we carefully look to help them describe, express and organize their thoughts and feelings. So, we may begin to "put words to experience" for them. We do this carefully, keeping in mind if the patient allows us to be

a placeholder for their agency and authority, we do not do so as experts who know what the solution is for symptoms much less their life dilemma. The agency or authority we exercise, then, is done in the service of creating the space and for securing time for the patient to resume their own search for a solution.

4   Lastly, we try also to imagine the questions that our patients would ask us and the statements they would make from this position *if* language and agency were more presently available to them. We try to mentalize not just their experiences outside the room but also inside the room and so imagine what they could be curious about. We imagine, for instance, the internal, unconscious dialogue of the patient to be: (A) This immersion feels like my "rightful destiny" and yet I'm still unsettled. Why? (B) What happens if I leave this immersion? I fear I will be overwhelmed in feelings of loss and confusion. I'm clinging but "what if I let go?" (C) I want your help but are you going to push me beyond what I can tolerate?

Sitting with patients in the paranoid-schizoid position

When we are in the paranoid-schizoid position we operate out of fear that our "bad" parts will be met with retaliation on the part of our caretakers who we are dependent upon to have our needs to be met. Accordingly, as we depict more in Chapters 5 (suicide) and 6 (otherness), the hallmarks of the paranoid-schizoid position entail the dual operations of "splitting" and "projection." These basic defenses are how small children deal with their anxieties that their "badness" will prevent them from getting their needs met. In their first encounter with otherness, with the feeling of dread caused from the incongruity of recognizing that their parent cannot possibly attend to their every need, the child begins to organize their world into terms of "good" and "bad." This splitting into a binary view is a result of projecting the "bad" feelings into the other – or part of the other – so as to preserve the feelings of goodness.

Semiotically, what we see happening here is as follows. The child begins to represent their experience of "me" and "not-me." In order, for the "me" (A) to be devoid of anxiety, the other or "not-me" (non-A) must be the "bad" one. This then is the first transformation of the non-A field. As a result, the child learns that non-A or "non-me" is "bad" in order for "me" to be good. Notably, the child's lack of perspective limits the "bad" to parts of the non-me. So, when the parent can metabolize the "bad" feelings that have been put into them by the child, they can return the projections in more tolerable (less anxiety-inducing) forms.

The embodiment of this might be exemplified, for instance, in a parent conveying to their child, "I know you are hungry and want to be fed now but it's going to take a minute for the bottle to warm. It can be hard to wait." Through doing this, the "bad" non-me becomes open to further transformation for the child such that they do not have to be "all bad," eventually paving the way to more depressive functioning. However, this takes quite a bit of time, and when within the throes of the paranoid-schizoid position, we can become overwhelmed with dread that our "badness" will not be metabolized and that our needs will be "too much." Then, we fear various forms of retaliation that reflect a paranoid anxiety of being surrounded by harmful others. This, then, can devolve into schizoid tendencies wherein we seek distance from this anxiety by seeking isolation from relationships.

If, for whatever reason, we become stuck within this level of being-ness, we function as persons "hungry for the desirable deserter" (Guntrip, 1968, p. 25). We are starving for the other all the while suspecting that they will "desert" us and so leave our needs unmet our desires unsatisfied. Of course, this turns the other into an existential threat, holding out both our salvation and also our destruction. We deal with this by turning the other into a "not-me," so that our "me" is protected from feelings of "badness." Instead, "not-me" becomes the "bad" one so that we can be (remain) "good" and have some hope of receiving our just desserts.

Patients in the paranoid-schizoid position, then, are more able to formulate experience (Stern, 2009) but are inclined to do so in more rigid and concrete ways which reflect relating to self and other in simplistic black and white terms. While there is more differentiation of self and other, the experience resides mostly as "me" and "not me" with an emphasis on whether the "not me" here is seeing "me" as "good" or "bad." Persons in the paranoid-schizoid position want the others in their life to view them as "all good" and act in ways to promote this praise or to disavow (defensively) its importance.

Thus, within the paranoid-schizoid position, there is more range of motion for otherness than in the contiguous position, but this range is subject to fields that become hyper-regulated such that freedom for meaning-making is highly delimited. Consequently, we as the therapist might find ourselves judging the patient, being pulled to praise the patient, or overly fixated upon whether they like the patient and vice versa. In these situations, the patient often presents their experience in ways that draws out an impassioned response from the therapist with either a challenging or affirming cast. The patient wants the therapist "on their side" and frustration of this is deeply felt as a threat to their being-ness. Hence, freedom to explore new meaning is constrained with the always present need to weave it into an affirmation of the worthiness of what already prevails.

In other words, in the patient's concern about how they are perceived, there is little tolerance for a grayness that reflects a mixture of "good" and "bad." Moreover, there is not a lot of room for curiosity about other self-states beyond the "good and the bad." In this regard, a key aspect of treatment is to consider a patient's conduct within this position as perhaps reflective of an as yet unformulated self-state looking for expression in what feels like a hostile territory.

And, indeed, there is hostility and anger within the paranoid-schizoid position. The patient often feels thwarted not only in the affirmation of their me-ness but also in the fledgling expression of themselves that might go beyond the limits inherent to their preliminary sense of individuation. Hence, they can feel as if they are living for someone else. This someone does not need to be external (i.e., mother or father) but may be a demanding and aggressive self-state that demands "perfection" and "excellence" and which insists that they always "know" how to do "the right thing." Thus, it is not uncommon to hear of "imposter syndrome" as reflective of other self-states who are impossible to silence because they represent an internalized demanding self-state that cannot be satisfied.

When within the paranoid-schizoid position the patient does not meet these impossibly high needs, there are tendencies to attack aggressively the self or other. We note in our work that usually the attacks start against oneself. This is because, in this position, the patient has not learned in a substantial way that their anger and rage can be safely expressed in the context of a relationship with another person. Instead, they fear the destructive capacities of their emotions, and they either turn that rage upon themselves for being insufficient for the achievement of greater one-ness with the desirable deserter or they defend against this by turning the rage toward "not-me's," who in paranoid fashion they view as thwarting their happy return to a contiguous one-ness.

In the first of these two reactions, they themselves are a "safe" target for the relentless nature of these attacks. The experience of being a "piece of shit," "utterly worthless," a "failure who will not amount to anything" is intense. In the second reaction, the vitriol toward the thwarting not-me's can be equally merciless. Both of these reactions can reflect either the anxieties of parental figures or the internalized version of these parental figure's own paranoid-schizoid self-states. However, we note that the ability to attack the "other" in some capacity rather than only one's self might also be thought of as an important, developmental progression toward eventually achieving the depressive position.

Working clinically with patients in the paranoid-schizoid position

Our work as therapists with these patients, then, is complicated. It entails initially joining the patient and working on the basis of limited self-object relationships. If all goes well, slowly and over considerable time, it is possible to begin introducing the subjectivity of otherness to the patient. This entails moving from self-object to self-other re-lating. In this respect, we hold in mind that the patient is straddling a wish to be affirmed as a "good me" worthy of "one-ness" *and* also a wish to escape the delimitation of only "good" or "bad" so that more nuanced iterations of their being can emerge. In the frustration that is inherent to this straddled position, they feel either the rage at themselves for being unworthy or rage at others for denying them the affirmation due to them. Hence, the introduction of the therapist's subjectivity runs the risk of either being experienced as either "friend or foe," something to be either sought or fought against.

Working with these patients entails an elaboration of this aggres-sion, which is either being externalized or internalized. It entails the need to help them and others (often the therapist) to "survive" the aggression so that it can be integrated back within the self-system. This process involves a blend of carefully increased subjectivity, either of the analyst but also of others in the patient's life so that the patient can begin to consider the effect their aggression has on themselves and others. The questions we promote in the therapy are then of the phenomenological and relational. They are ones wherein therapist wonders with patient about how other people view them and how they think they are coming across.

In helping patient to elaborate this aggression, it is important to note that a frequent countertransference reaction is to falter in our willingness to bring this aggression into the therapy relationship itself. If we join the patient in "splitting," we fall into a collusion with seeing the "bad" people as being "out there." In doing this, we can easily mistake simple expression of the aggression with integration of it. Bringing the aggression into the room, of course, often can take some doing as the patient hopes to preserve the "goodness" of the therapist and so of themselves. Nevertheless, it is crucial that we do so. True progress, of course, is when the anger is contained *within and not pushed out* of the therapy relationship. When it is pushed out, we are simply preserving the "me/not-me" position by substituting one that is "us/not-us."

Thus, in situating ourselves and our questions we do so with a deep appreciation of the existential threat that our *difference* or otherness makes to the patient. There is no understatement entailed in saying that any expression of our otherness entails an important measure of being experienced as either "the desirable deserter" who won't affirm their being a "good" one or "the hateful robber" who seeks to take away their being the "good" one and make them a "bad" one (Guntrip, 1968, p. 25).

In this, patients within the paranoid-schizoid position can come across as an infuriating mixture of both help-seeking and help-rejecting, as they seek affirmation of their feelings of entitlement. In treating others essentially as objects, who exist only as a "not-me" and who are only permitted to see certain aspects of "me," the patient in the paranoid-schizoid position demands a certain type of response and rejects most others. Thus, a challenge is to understand the need for a patient to hold certain views and how this has been protective for them in the past. Firmness and a willingness to be experienced as the objectification of these unsavory personifications, inevitably, will feel unjust. But expecting "justice" in how we are treated as a therapist is not realistic if we are going to meaningfully engage our patients. Expectedly then, a great deal of patience, courage to be vulnerable to attack and perspective on the part of the therapist are required for the work to bear fruit.

It is important to not overlook this as patients within their paranoid-schizoid position sometimes function at very high levels. Their demanding self-structure can draw out truly impressive accomplishments that both maintain the vicious feedback cycle but also convince them that it is working. There is a sense of precariousness here that if they break from it, they could collapse back toward a contiguous position. In fact, sometimes this collapse "back" is necessary. This does not have to be seen as regressive but rather as something which allows for self-states that had been neglected and restrained from coming forth to "speak."

Approach and questions in the paranoid-schizoid position

Here are some questions and perspectives we think typify work and functioning in the paranoid-schizoid position:

1   From the therapist's perspective, our questions center around how much otherness our clients are able to tolerate. In this, efforts at inquiry are aimed at helping to explicate how and why patients are experiencing the world in the terms and ways that they are. This involves a willingness to look at the relationships but not necessarily immediately challenge and express alternative perspectives, especially if we do not think they can tolerate much otherness. At this point, the questions, we might ask them, instead, to describe "How they have come to see things this way?" Or, "What would happen if we looked at things in this way?" Similarly, we might inquire about ways they have felt their goodness to have been unseen or what happened when they were bad.

2   As we begin to introduce otherness, we can do so with an emphasis on part/whole relationships. So, we might ask if part of

them feels one way and part another way. Similarly, we might be curious if their way of seeing it is 100% or do they think some of them see it differently. If we think that they can tolerate more otherness, we might wonder what it would be like if we asked something like, "how do you think others perceive that?" Similarly, we might ask, "I wonder if you think this way about me?"

3   From the patient's perspective, some questions we may imagine them thinking (consciously or unconsciously) are: "Are you with me or against me? Do you see how special my me-ness is? Can you really be with me (love me) if you are seeing something other than this specialness to which I cling? How might I survive giving up my way of being in the world?"

Depressive positioning

When patients present in the depressive position or when they move from paranoid-schizoid position into depressive positioning within a session, there may be a concern for how their actions affected other people or an effort to grapple with the limitations in how they view themselves. Thus, in the depressive position, patients are able to consider various aspects of themselves and others with greater openness and curiosity but also with considerable anxiety and fear about how their and other's worthiness will be evaluated. They can tolerate more detailed inquiry into their narratives and sustain the therapist's attempts to deconstruct the narrative.

Here, then, a certain aspect of the depressive position is the necessary "loss" we experience in knowing who we and who others are. In the face of this loss, we need to be able to tolerate/embrace the reappraisal of our sense of others and our self, but especially our self. Holding this "loss" out of reach from the persecutory judgment that characterizes the paranoid-schizoid binary frame of "either good or bad" can be difficult and so entry into the depressive position may be challenged by our retreat into a "manic defense." Here, we feel unable to tolerate protracted reflection and feel, instead, a heightened urgency immediately and definitively to redefine ourselves, often through actions, in ways that we think will cast us as "still a good person" who has not "lost" anything. In short, when we enter into the depressive position and so begin to come to terms with the limits that effect all of us, our sense of self and our feeling of belonging is threatened, and we can sometimes seek to short-circuit our immersion in this disjunction by grasping quickly onto new conjunction.

Notably, this defense, unlike the dominating defenses of the paranoid-schizoid position, is in some ways more easily observed and interpreted. As it is a reaction to loss, the defense implicitly marks that that loss at least preconsciously is being acknowledged. We can consider, then, that the manic defense is a kind of weigh station in the journey toward the new existential situated-ness that comes with meeting the challenges of the depressive position.

Of course, the challenges of the depressive position generate considerable tensions. On the one hand, we look at patterns of how we relate to self and others in our life with more freedom from the anxious binary of the paranoid-schizoid position. On the other hand, our growing awareness of the possibilities of difference and for being different can overwhelm us. We have to grapple with guilt and anxiety at how we were and whether in being this way we have caused harm. In this, we yield some of the schizoid defense we might have held when we were convinced that we needed to exist independent of others to maintain our sense of being-ness. Rather, in the depressive position, we come to recognize that our sense of being is contingent upon other people, especially those whom we feel we have harmed and with whom we need to reconcile and make repair. In this effort, we hope that others recognize their own humanity and so treat ours with grace.

However, when we are here working toward new anchoring, "being at sea" can consume us in a fear that makes at least partial retreat to the known paranoid-schizoid harbor seem like a way of preserving valued aspects of ourselves. New "naming's" requires "un-naming" and that, in short, can be unhinging. We can devolve into a fear that we will lose ourselves during the process and not find our way back (into a new conjunction). Similarly, we worry that we may lose the positive and loving appraisals of our being that we have imagined people have of us. Tolerating that we can be both loved and admired but also frustrating can be hard and scary, especially when being in the depressive position may entail certain "naming's" about ourselves that important others may find disconcerting or threatening to their own stability.

Too much of this fear and concern about how we and others see us may generate an obsessional type of defense (Sullivan, 1956). Here, the patient appears to have a solid grasp on self and other, but is, in fact, constantly in suspense about whether their "hatefulness" casts them irretrievably as unforgivable destroyers. Their manifest deliberation about whether things are really "as they should be" or "right and correct" rests on a looping, subtextual inner conversation about whether they and others are "good" (which is the paranoid-schizoid "coloring" of this) or "reliably loving and caring" (which is the depressive coloring for which they are reaching).

Often, then, concern about how our patients' being is impacting other people can strike us initially as appropriately self-reflective and self-conscientious. However, their stumbling ability to move from thinking to embodied action and their deep level of concern of how they are seen belies this. They can become obsessed with impression management which leads ultimately to being stuck in the false self "solution" that Winnicott (1960) notes. This is a solution that sits on the border of paranoid-schizoid and depressive positioning. The awareness of self and other are more reflective about depressive sensibilities, but the anxieties of agency and the inability to ground subjectivity more fully reflects the sticky grasp of the paranoid-schizoid position. This can create a tricky blend to work with as much remains disguised due to the patients abiding fear of authenticity.

Working clinically in the depressive position

In navigating these waters, the therapist can be helped in the work by the greater range of freedom they have for the expression of their own subjectivity. Since our being is less threatening to the patient's sense of self, we are able to work with the patients in ways which more fully reflect our experiences of being a self with the patient. From this perspective, our questions are more of a self-other nature. While this, of course, can happen also within the paranoid-schizoid and even contiguous positions since patients in the depressive position are often concerned about their effect on others, we become a useful and important other for this focus.

As the therapist here we can be both the *subjective other* who makes use of their own experiences with the patient but also the *objective other* who imagines how the patient's agency may come across to people outside of the room. Indeed, with the depressive position, we are able to tolerate better the sometimes clumsy and anxiety-riddled attempts of the patient's self-aggression and, thereby, to make room for our de-authorization as any misconstrued font of ultimate truth. Thus, for patients whose parents were not able to tolerate the patient's evolution into greater being-ness, in the depressive position we as therapists can play an important role in validating and authorizing the patient's burgeoning understanding of agency while working simultaneously to provide space for the deconstruction of external authority. All of this, of course, involves the patient having the foundation with us to trust that we will survive their aggression.

As this foundation extends and the patient's fear of being an unforgivable destroyer recedes, patients are able to straddle less urgently and hold more consistently the depressive position. In doing so they can begin better to make connections to the early relational and attachment experiences which induced their paranoid-schizoid ways of being. Within the depressive position, patients are thus able to identify their own pitfalls, triggers and anxieties that may undermine their ability to fluidly "be" in the world. Thus, much of what has been termed "working through" occurs within the depressive position.

A key aspect of our work within the depressive position with adolescents hinges on our understanding that without adequate time and space for this "working through" of "how" they have journeyed into their being-ness, they are more susceptible later in life to defensive organizations that reflect devolution into the earlier "solutions" to being which characterize the paranoid-schizoid and contiguous positions. This time and space is increasingly a privilege that many college students and counseling centers do not have, and in recognition of this shortfall of resource and time and often when reflecting with a student about our work together, we will in a glancing way acknowledge this by saying some version of one or both of the following statements: (1) "I hope that when you [student] look back on our conversations you will say to yourself: 'That was OK; it was good to talk to him [Philip or Rick]. I could do this again with someone [a therapist] if I feel somehow stuck again" and/or (2) "I hope you [student] will hold fast to the idea that we are all an evolving story. Each chapter that we write recasts the previous ones, and sometimes in life we are called upon at one point more than another to consider what we've written and what we *are* presently writing."

The increased demands upon college counseling centers that are often not closely matched by increased supply of clinical hours and so the ever-growing reliance upon models of treatment that are shorter term or more structured, means that students do not get to "work through" aspects of themselves. Thus, while these interventions may be helpful at moving students from paranoid-schizoid to depressive position, without a more thorough understanding we think students are susceptible to sliding backward, often without the tools needed to marshal back toward the depressive position. Indeed, for some students for whom compliance and self-authorization remain issues, these more structured interventions risk substituting their experience of themselves as agentic with a false compliance with authority.

Approach and questions in the depressive position

Our approach to questions that we may ask and consider our patients asking of us focusing here on their greater capacities for symbolization and meaning-making and to tolerate inquiry.

1   In working with the depressive position, we focus on what the patient imagines the experience of others (including us) to be in a particular instance. Thus, we might ask directly about how they think we as the therapist experienced or might react to something that they said. When patients are in the depressive position, we may also be more willing to disclose our own reactions, especially those that perhaps feel far afield. Accordingly, we may say something like, "Do you mind if I share my association to what you've said?"

2   Similarly, we can also challenge patients with greater freedom when they are in the depressive position. We can say things along the lines of "I'm aware that you want to express aspects of yourself that you feel others will have trouble accepting." In challenging, we do not hope to "undermine" our patient's agency and self but rather to suggest to them that things can be

complicated in their many sided-ness. We try to embrace in our words and by our demeanor our conviction that with deconstruction of who we (both the client and therapist) are can come fresh and creative new reconstruction.

3   On our patient's side, the depressive position may manifest with more conscious concern about what the therapist thinks of them. This can be reflected in difficulties speaking or doing so with an eye toward impression management. The patient may think that the therapist will judge them or look down upon them once they see their "lack" or "badness." Thus, they may feel like the therapist is not someone who can get it or seek to ascertain that the therapist understands shame and guilt.

Transcendent position

Notably, patients rarely present themselves to us in the transcendent position. This makes sense as it is from this position that we are able to live in a way that embraces curiosity, discovery and openness. This does not mean, however, that we do not get to work with patients in this position or that it cannot be achieved within the context of a therapeutic relationship. Rather, this is often the reward for extended periods of hard work and can represent gratifying experiences for therapist and patient. We are reminded here of Winnicott's quips about how at the end of an analysis that the analyst can share with the patient just how hard the work was and they can enjoy the ways that the patient was in fact difficult. Moreover, just because we achieve this position does not mean we hold it stably and that our work may be done around the movement to and from it. In this regard, we think that patients in the transcendent position often present with a request for consultation be-cause in reference to some event or conundrum they recognize that they have mislaid their grasp on the "radically dialogic" nature of truth (Felman, 1985, p. 125). They sense that they are speaking past their otherness to themselves (and, therefore, the otherness of others), that they, at least for the present time, are having trouble representing the "dialogue" within themselves and, therefore, need the live embrace that comes with talking *in situ* with a trusted other.

For what we hope might be a fitting capstone to the ideas of this chapter and also as way of portraying what we understand the consultation question of the person in the transcendent position to be, we offer a somewhat light in spirit image for consideration. It is an image that we came upon when we prepared a publication about the subject of resilience (Webb & Rosenbaum, 2019). Ahead of sharing this image, we ask the reader as they proceed to hold in mind our conclusion about consultation in the transcendent position: the patient is *looking for help in changing "seats."*

We invite the readers to put themselves in Plato's (c. 375 BCE/ 1918) cave. This is the cave that many of us first encounter in a philosophy course. It is the cave which Plato uses to characterize how we are constrained in life in our access to truth. We are all in the cave together, we can only see a version of Truth as a shadow on the wall before us. This shadow representation is cast by the light of a torch (the "projector") that lies out of sight behind and inaccessible to us.

We extend Plato's story in a way that we're not certain conforms with his notions but we think aptly suits explication of the contiguous, paranoid-schizoid, depressive and transcendent positions. In the cave, much as in a theater, there are different places to sit and each has its own unique perspective.

In the autistic-contiguous "seat," we don't realize we are in a cave or that there is something to be observed.

In the paranoid-schizoid position we know we are in the cave looking at the wall, but we don't know that what's before us is only a shadow. Furthermore, we assume that our "seat" or row is the best one for seeing truth.

In the depressive position, it dawns on us that we see on the wall is a representation, a semblance of truth. We begin to grasp that this representation is gray; afterall, it's a shadow. We begin to understand that the seats of others for viewing it offer different angles and, thereby, relative advantages and disadvantages.

Lastly, in the transcendent stage, we embrace that seats for viewing the shadow of truth offer different views on its distortion but that our chance for best approximation and consideration of truth, despite the inevitable distortions, is to gather in as many perspectives on it as possible. The old adage about the sum being equal to more than the sum of its parts applies, and we set out to see how we can negotiate our freedom to change seats frequently, even in a disciplined way.

References

Felman, S (1985). *Jacques Lacan and the adventure of insight*. Harvard University Press.

Grossmark, R (2018). *The Unobtrusive Relational Analyst*. New York: Routledge.

Guntrip, H (1968). *Schizoid phenomena, object-relations, and the self*. International Universities Press.

Marková, I (2003a). *Dialogicality and social representations*. Cambridge, UK: Cambridge University Press.

Marková, I (2003b). Constitution of the self: Intersubjectivity and dialogicality. *Culture & Psychology, 9* (3), 249–259. 10.1177/1354067X030093006

Peirce, CP (1965). *The collected papers of Charles Sanders Peirce, V. 1–6* (C Hartshorne C., & P Weiss P., Eds.), *V. 7* (A Burks. Ed.). Harvard University Press.

Plato. (1918). *The Republic of Plato* (A Kerr, Trans).https://www.google.com/books/edition/The_Republic_of_Plato/JSFQAQAAIAAJ?hl=en&gbpv=1&pg=PR1&printsec=frontcover (Original work c. 375 BCE)

Quillman, T (2012). Neuroscience and therapist self-disclosure. Deepening right brain to right brain communication between therapist and patient. *Clinical Social Work Journal, 40* (1), 1–9. DOI 10.1007/s10615-011-0315-8

Schore, JR & Schore, AN (2008). Modern attachment theory: The central role of affect regulation in development and treatment. *Clinical Social Work Journal, 36* (1), 9–20. DOI: 10.1007/s10615-007-0111-7

Stern, DB (2006). Opening what has been closed, relaxing what has been clenched: Dissociation and enactment over time in committed relationships. *Psychoanalytic Dialogues, 16* (6), 747–761. 10.1080/10481880701357446

Stern, DB (2009). *Partners in Thought: Working with Unformulated Experience, Dissociation and Enactment*. Routledge Publications.

Stern, DB (2015). *Relational Freedom: Emergent Properties of the Interpersonal Fields*. Routledge Publications.

Sullivan, HS (1956). *Clinical studies in psychiatry*. W.W. Norton.

Webb, RE & Rosenbaum, P (2019). Resilience and thinking perpendicularly: A meditation or morning jog? *Journal of College Student Psychotherapy, 33* (1). Advance online publication. 10.1080/87568225.2018.1449687.

Winnicott, DW (1960). Ego distortion in terms of true and false self. In *The maturation process and the facilitating environment* (pp. 140–157). International Universities Press.

Chapter 4

Appreciating "Destructive" Processes in Adolescence[1]

D.W. Winnicott's consideration of destruction

The role of destruction during the developmental processes leading to the emergence of a separate sense of self has long been a topic of discussion. For example, as alluded to in Chapter 2, D.W. Winnicott viewed the destruction of the object as well as its survival of this destruction as crucial in the movement from object relating toward object usage. In his paper "The use of an object and relating through identification," he writes:

> A new feature thus arrives in the theory of object-relating [as it evolves into object-usage]. The subject says to the object: 'I destroyed you,' and the object is there to receive the communication. From now on the subject says: 'Hullo object!' 'I destroyed you.' 'I love you.' 'You have value for me because of your survival of my destruction of you.' 'While I am loving you I am all the time destroying you in (unconscious) *fantasy*.' (1971, p. 90)

Slowing this down, for Winnicott infants begin their lives by relating to objects primarily within their inner world. Possessing limited (albeit also sophisticated) capacities for relating, he theorizes that infants relate to mother primarily internally. As we discussed in Chapters 1 and 2, they project who they are into mother who returns these projections as best as she can, creating a feeling of continuity, linearity and togetherness. Object-relating thus assumes a shared reality and the feelings of sameness and continuity.

DOI: 10.4324/9781003246558-5

While necessary for the infant to feel safe and secure, object-relating has to give way to the more sophisticated form of object usage. The capacity to "use" objects speaks to their existence outside of the infant's inner world. It is their very existence as outside of the infant that lets the infant use them. For Winnicott (1969), "destruction turns up" (p. 91) or occurs as a normal and situational result of the child's increasingly complex needs not being met by their M-other. These experiences generate experiences of frustration and are the onset of the recognition of separateness and difference. The baby's experience is no longer contiguous with M-other. Out of anger, frustration and fear, the baby in their fantasy destroys M-other (sometimes these fantasies can also be seen in reality, such as times babies bite the breast and toddlers delight in crumbling block towers). This serves to both locate their anger outside of them in an object so that they do not have to view themselves as bad.

Simultaneously, that there is an object to destroy that exists outside of them creates the transition or bridge between the baby's inner world to the outer world, which generates a sense of exteriority for the baby/infant in contrast to interiority. If the object/M-other can survive this destruction, by which Winnicott means continue to function as a dependable Other who does not retaliate and so continues to meet the baby's needs, the child then (re)internalizes them. The experience moves to unconscious memory, where they can continually destroy and recreate M-other as they work to gain control over inner and outer experiences.

Achieving object usage signals the introduction and tolerance of difference. In object usage, we learn to enjoy the otherness of the subject in addition to our sameness. This paves the way for later interpersonal connection, experiences of agency and deeper relating.

More recent readings

The central and enduring question, then, that Winnicott tackles is: How do we become subjects in the world who can appreciate limits and boundaries around our own subjectivity and agency as well as that of Others? Winnicott's views are taken up again in an important paper by Thomas Ogden (2016). In this paper, titled "Destruction reconceived: On Winnicott's 'The use of an object and relating through identifications,'" Ogden reconsiders Winnicott's way of understanding surviving destructive attacks.

Specifically, Ogden argues that Winnicott's reading does not create enough room for the M-other to experience and acknowledge feelings of real hurt and destruction. He writes that the process of moving from object relating to usage centers on "the reality that something important about the mother's experience of herself (and the infant's experience of her) as a mother is actually destroyed" (Ogden, 2016, p. 1250). What Ogden notably thinks is destroyed is M-other's feelings of themselves as "good enough." Toward this end, Ogden writes:

> The destruction of the mother's experience of herself as mother may take innumerable forms, for instance by her coming to feel as if she is not fit to be a mother because she is unable to console her baby when he is in terrible distress, or is not sufficiently loving for the infant to nurse at the breast, or unable to help her infant sleep when he is so desperately in need of sleep, or hating her baby for keeping her from all the pleasures and sources of pride and competence and creativity that she had in her life before the baby was born, or any thousand other ways an infant and child may actually destroy his mother's belief in her adequacy as mother (and, at times, her adequacy as a worthwhile person of any sort). (p. 1250)

Note that the examples offered above are all situational. Destruction emerges as a result of a baby/infant being a baby/infant and not out of any premeditated motivation or unconcious instinct to attack or destroy. Rather, the baby's unceasing needs (expressed or experienced as demands) inevitably lead to mother's faltering. The infant responds to the inevitable failure of the M-other to meet all of their increasingly complex needs and desires in ways that challenge the M-other's ability to conceptualize themselves as "good." In a felt and real way (not fantasied), M-other experiences and so feels some of themselves, particularly their identity as a M-other as being destroyed. And yet, since destruction turns up, this is destruction without a destroyer. It is crucial that M-other recognize this, for if they consider their baby as actively destroying them, then they are locating the destructive agency within the baby and not the situation out of which the destruction turns up.

Thus, we may say that for both Ogden and Winnicott, the baby's destructive actions occur in the realm of fantasy. There is no agency or intentionality on the part of the baby, their destruction emerges as a reflex to certain inevitable experience. However, for Ogden, unlike Winnicott, M-other's experience is of being destroyed in reality. This creates or identifies an asymmetry. If M-other feels and is in fact destroyed by their baby they have to deal with what can be an overwhelming wash of real emotions that emerge from their destruction. They cannot in other words leave their own destruction to the realm of the baby's fantasy or treat it as an "as if" experience. It is real and they need to deal with it as such.

Since these events are real, as marked by M-other's experience and feelings of pain and destruction, their child's empathic attunement to them and then successful tolerance of them are crucial. These feelings are communicated, consciously or unconsciously to the infant, who senses, experiences and responds to M-other's felt hurt and pain. It is essential that the M-other be able to survive the destruction that is at hand; they have to experience being destroyed without being "killed." In regulating their feelings in a "good enough" fashion caregivers manage and tolerate the pain of this destruction and forebear from retaliatory responses. When "killed," they totally cease functioning as a caregiver.

M-other's "good enough" self-regulation helps the infant to manage the pain experienced in sympathetic connection to them and, thereby, allows the infant to learn to regulate their own emotions. This is a critical developmental moment for the infant since in a fundamental way the infant's existence hinges on the outcome of this dynamic exchange with the M-other. If M-others cannot manage their feelings, they can unwittingly overwhelm the infant with their own experience. It is through this linkage between the M-other being destroyed, as only a real person can, and the infant feeling both the M-other's pain and their survival that the infant moves from relating to usage.

The question of agency

In our own reading of Ogden (Rosenbaum & Webb, 2021), we take up what we see as the questionable misapplication of agency. While both Ogden and Winnicott are clear that destruction turns up – that it is not a result of intention, we think their explication of this developmental process remains ambiguous with respect to the questions of destruction and agency. While they might argue that it is exactly this ambiguity that is necessary for the transitional space by which interiority and exteriority are created, we consider it unnecessarily problematic.

From our perspective, the ambiguity and misapplication of agency are structural. It comes along when we link destruction with the intersection of creation. In other words, to talk about destruction and creation as necessary for development is to invite a confusing conversation about the role of agency regardless of how insistent we are that "destruction turns up." We consider this confusion and as reflecting the ways both Winnicott and Ogden are trying to reconcile themselves to the semiotic grounds or legacy of Melanie Klein, who herself is dealing with Freud's legacy. As such, both Winnicott and Ogden are committed to holding and modifying Klein's view that the infant dwells in a stormy unconscious instinctual world in reaction to their encounter with reality (Klein, 1975a, 1975b). That the destructive agency is intrinsic to the baby's unconscious experience. They are in other words straddling what they know and assert – that destruction turns up – with a historical legacy that asserts that the baby's unconscious is agentically destructive.

Not breaking away from this historical legacy in a clear way hinders the development of theory that can grapple with the crucial questions of how agency and subjectivity develop in the lap of destruction without falling into a muddiness, which invites a misapplication of agency to the child. In other words, even when we are clear that destruction turns up, once we've considered destruction of the parent as *essential* (as *required* for the development of subjectivity), we have to grapple with whether or not the infant intends to cause hurt. While it can be argued that the ambiguity of this intent is a challenge that a M-other might experience and need to survive, we are not convinced that clinical theory is well-served by either sustaining this ambiguity or making attributions of infant agency that stretch commonsense.

It was this conviction that led to our development of an alternative analogy for viewing this parent-child interaction and the emergence of agency and object usage. This analogy (first noted in Chapter 1) is drawn from physics. Recall that physics considers the duality of subatomic matter and considers its essence to be simultaneously that of being a wave and particle. As has now been long established by quantum physicists, a "gaggle" of subatomic matter travels as a wave, as a potentiality, until it "collapses" into a locatable "particle" when it is "observed" (or "measured").[2]

We found this understanding analogously useful for considering what happens in the development of personhood and in the concomitant evolution of an appreciation of otherness. It is apt to say that we as persons are a kind of "gaggle" of matter and that we start out our lives with a broad wave of potential self-states and identities. Over time our potential delimits itself as we are "measured" or positioned in culture and language by ourselves and by others. Our identities reflect the complicated history of how our wave of potential being-ness has been serially "collapsed" into articulation by language, by naming.

In other words, there is a tension between our being able to travel as a wave of potential and the times when we are necessarily (or not) "collapsed" by others into locatable particles. These "collapses" in turn influence the "wave" of our being in ways that begin to restrict and enable certain identities to form. Moreover, the process of how this occurs, whether it is done with our burgeoning selves in mind and lightly held or done with strict and demanding constraints, which includes societal structuring greatly informs how we go about exploring our potentials at later points in life. Joshua Rothman captures beautifully much of the essence of this, remarking:

> We all dwell in the here and now; we all have actual selves, actual lives. But what are they? Selves and lives have penumbras and possibilities – that's what's unique about them. They are always changing, and so are always new; they refuse to stand still. We live in anticipation of their meaning, which will inevitably exceed what can be known or said. (2020, p. 73)

Furthermore, we can approach destruction in a way which semiotically recasts it as an elaboration of the A <> non-A field. Whether it be the breast to feed the child or language to name our world, once we recognize that the introduction of *anything* brings with it a relationship to what *it* is not, we are not contingent upon destruction to create the external world. The tension between breast <> non-breast or inner world <> non-inner world exists axiomatically even if, at first, it can only be consciously "known" by the parent. This knowing, however, structures the relational field between parent and baby such that the baby's experiences can be an elaboration of A, into "good" breast (A^1) "bad breast" (A^2) and so forth. Thus, "good" and "bad" are not separate fields but instead linked elaborations of an experience. Similarly, the possibility of non-breast or discontinuous experience already exists in the process of feeding such that it is not necessary to postulate its creation.

Thus, moving from object relating or contiguous experience to usage involves the baby's burgeoning ability both to explore the realm of A but also move as a wave through non-A and not be particularized in punitive ways by M-other. Destruction in other words is not needed to conceptualize how the baby creates reality, since the relationship exists *a priori* within the matrix and attachment to M-other. Instead, we can shift the experience of real destruction to later childhood and adolescence where there can be more of a shared reality (object usage).

Killing without murder: Adolescence and later childhood and the multiplicity of selves

So, what does it mean then for us to relocate "real destruction" to later childhood and adolescence? We can just imagine here the quips of readers who are parents, especially of adolescents. In fact, in what follows we will focus primarily on adolescents because in adolescence the "killing without murder" is most dramatically evident. We recognize, however, that later-aged children show early versions of what the adolescent embodies and that even as adults we might destroy and kill without murder. One of Winnicott's more notable examples of the issue of the child seeking "proof of his guardian's ability to hate objectively" (1975, p. 199) in the face of destructive actions by the child is about a nine-year-old boy.

Differences between destruction with intent, killing and murdering

To get to the process of "killing without murder" and "destruction with intent," it is important to consider the context within which it

occurs: adolescents' and later-aged children's seemingly contradictory and paradoxical conduct. Having said this, we hasten to say
that what seems chaotic, disruptive, destructive and irrational to
adults contains the potential for constructive elaboration of ways of
relating to self and other. Accordingly, while adolescents may also
feel chaotic and irrational much of their experience may also feel
normal and may make complete sense to them even if they cannot
always articulate "why." This may be one of the reasons contemporary psychoanalytic theories that eschew the singular, isolated
and integrated self in favor of a network of related but discrete self-
states seem to make so much sense in our work with young people
(see Chapter 6 for an elaboration of these theories).

The first place these theories help us is in understanding how
adolescents and later-aged children "kill without murdering" and
"destroy with intent." Here, we think that destruction involves the
real killing off of self-states of both parent and child. Recall from
earlier that we distinguished killing from destruction through the loss
of function. The parent (and therapist we might add) are "killed off"
when they cannot function in their role. So, in adolescence, the experience of killing might entail, for instance, the adolescent acting in
ways to kill the parent as their primary caretaker, instead preferring a
friend's parent, a peer or trusted teacher. The parent, in turn, may let
the adolescent know of their feelings of real hurt at losing this role.
This in turn may get elaborated into killing off their adolescent's
child-selves through now expecting certain behaviors, such as re-
sponsibilities, chores and particular ways of acting. Accordingly,
destruction is not entirely literal, i.e., it does not always entail destroying materials or one's physical self (though it can). As elaborated below, destruction is ideally only partial with both parties but
especially the parent maintaining other self-states from which to respond.

Emblematic of this is the interaction between the adolescent and
parent where we see the seemingly ubiquitous adolescent proclama-
tion to the parent of: "I hate you. Why can't you be like Charlie's
mother?"; and the admixture of anger and deep sadness in the parent's response: "What am I? Chopped liver? Go. Go ahead and cry
and laugh it up with Charlie's mother. Do what you want. You're
clearly going to do it regardless of what I say." Both parties have to

grapple with the fact that real selves are being "destroyed" (rarely, of course, is it so neat as being described).

What differentiates this destruction and killing from murder is that the parent hopefully has other-selves accessible (i.e., through other relationships to possible partners, family, profession or friends) such that they can maintain balance enough, such that all of themselves is not "destroyed" rather than a singular self (functioning within a role). Such a capacity to shift self-states or perspectives may allow for modification of self, such that the parent can re-find themselves in relationship to their child, perhaps less as primary caretaker and more as a caring and supportive other.

This is crucial since a central task of adolescent is the creation and elaboration of a multitude of their own self-states such that with any luck, they too, are not destroyed by their parents. In the creation and elaboration of these self-states, the adolescent actively works to deauthorize and thus to kill off their parent's ability to define their "wave," their sense of themselves. As we described in Chapter 2, parents have to allow for this de-authorization. While they might not always do this willingly or even agreeably, they fundamentally must do it with an openness that acknowledges their child's growing semiotic capacities to construct and explore identity.

Constructing identity to embrace otherness

Thus, while this process of identity construction and exploration mimics some of early child imaginative play, the key difference is that during adolescence some of these iterations of self are actively played with in the material world rather than in the realm of fantasy. Adolescents partake in cultural and social objects and artifacts, and through doing, they identify with various Others, whether musicians, politicians and political parties, artists, athletes, authors, etc., sometimes strongly taking on these identities in dress, actions, behaviors and ideologies (Zittoun et al., 2003; Zittoun & Gillespie, 2015).[3] They dress differently, get tattoos, take up smoking, try alcohol and push the boundaries of the previously consensually validated realities, even of the physical world. All of this may feel chaotic and contradictory on the part of their adult others, who feel as if they are weathering various storms and their previously sweet child besieged by hormones, trends they do not understand, friends they may or may not like, and so forth.

Shifting selves and taking on new identities, while maddening to parents who yearn for calm and consistency, is perhaps the required actions toward more fully encountering and relating to otherness. It is the imaginative play of the childhood, but it is reinvigorated through others more fully embodied in reality, even if these realities can have stark consequences. As such, this entails an earnestness and potential seriousness that is different than the social play of children. Whereas later in life this might be conceived as more a mental activity (perspective-taking), for adolescents it is often not enough to consider something from someone else's perspective, they must first embody and occupy other perspectives. Through doing so, they may experience the need to hold these perspectives with certainty, demonstrating an ironic concreteness and similarity. (Think here of the old adage that all teenagers express their independence by dressing alike.)

In other words, the adolescent actively challenges if not destroys interpretations of who they are (both for themselves and others as well) in an ongoing process of exploration. In this regard, they may be seen as pushing back on being understood or named. Naming, of course, is tantamount to becoming locatable or "particularized." Jacques Lacan recognizes the aggression (and destruction) in naming … in speaking. He says, "All I can do is tell the truth. No, that isn't so – I have missed it. There is no truth that, in passing through awareness, does not lie. But one runs after it all the same" (1978, p. vii). Speaking to Lacan's perspective, Ogden says, "[T]he meanings we create through language are inevitably built upon misnamings, misrecognitions that we rely upon to create the illusion of understanding" (1992, p. 523).

Adolescents either implicitly or explicitly begin to play at the realization that to be recognized and named is to also in some sense to "lie" about having captured the essence of being-ness. This opens up tremendous areas of self-expression but can also cause doubts and anxieties. Thus, adolescents are often ambivalent about being understood or even understanding themselves. Understanding after all represents the collapse of the wave into a way of being at a time when their primary activity/interest is in expanding the wave in order to see who they want to be. Being "understood" may not be the warm embrace we imagine it to be later in life but rather a sense of being pinned or trapped into a way of being. The parent's relief at under-standing their adolescent is the adolescent's anxiety of feeling stuck.

What is required here from adults is not the passive weathering of the storm often associated with adolescent *sturm und drang* (Hall, 1904) but rather the active engagement in relating, making themselves available to be killed off in the manner to which Ogden points (Lacan, 1977). Parents, in other words, must work to find the dis-tance that allows them to let the child know that they are still there as a parent who appreciates them and their struggle for independence and that in this appreciation, they as a parent are working to re-calibrate how they situate themselves with respect to them as an adolescent. If the parent cannot engage but rather remains removed or if the parent struggles with finding balance such that they ex-perience the death of a self-state as a murder, then the adolescent loses out on important opportunities of seeing the effects of their agency on the world and on others. This can hinder their growth and experience of themselves as real agents in the world as well as their understanding about their ensuing impact on others.

With regards to the parent's inability to engage, the adolescent struggles to find an interlocutor with whom to lock horns with and define themselves relationally. Though this may take place elsewhere (such as with friends or teachers) the value of it occurring with the parent lies with the historical relationship of parent-child. In locking horns with the parents, the adolescent, as Ogden indicates, engages with both the parent and the parental representation of themselves (i.e., the adolescent). In this manner, destruction of parent and the adolescent's historical self takes place, paving the way for the re-construction of various self-states. Avoidance of this sends the mes-sage that the parent prefers the child to the adolescent and prevents recognition and acknowledgment of the adolescents burgeoning selves.

Alternatively, the parent's inability to survive destruction and so to be murdered (i.e., their own collapse of self-states into a singular self-state) is problematic because it saddles the adolescent with under-mining guilt and the need to make impossible reparation. In not being able to shift self-states and re-find their own balance, the parent also fixes the adolescent as a murderer. In turn, the adolescent sees both the killing of the parent and the loss of the entirety of the parent's sense of self as deadly rather than as just an important point in the evolution of their relationship to the parent. This deeply complicates the adolescent's experience of themselves as agentic causing them possibly to become inhibited and fearful of their agency.

During adolescence, then, we must destroy in order to separate and find our own destiny and different types of relating. Within the metaphor of quantum physics, we might say that we must destroy our relational gaggle of being that has particularized and seek re-potentiation of our wave of being-ness. If such agency for the budding adult being that an adolescent entails such consequential catastrophe, collapse into particularization, the bond of connection between the adolescent and the parent not only gets torn but also severed.

The adolescent's complicated quest for their agency can then result in a problematic retreat into a consumingly angry, depressed, or manic positioning of themselves in the world. We might then think that it is from here that increased physical destruction or attack upon themselves via cutting, burning or other risky conduct becomes seen. These "attacks upon the self" are often understood as expressions not only of psychic pain (Rosenbaum, 2016) but may also be seen as concrete forms of the destruction required for separation. At the most extreme, these attacks may result in suicidal crises, topics which we take up further in Chapter 5. Thus, in considering "self-harm," we need to not only consider the physical self of the adolescent but the relational self. The self-other relationship to caregivers and parents who have been involved in measuring and naming the adolescent.

We think that when parents can allow themselves to be de-authorized, when they can be killed without being murdered and when their multiplicity of being can surface despite the storm, the parent "parents" (themselves and the child); they help the adolescent find hope rather than danger in conflict. Perspective, empathy and role-taking become the order of the day. This, of course, can be difficult to achieve during the turbulence that this process can entail, especially when the threat manifests in physical or bodily expression. However, it is also simply that which is required for development to proceed.

Adolescents need to relate to similarity and difference in real ways. In this way, they both create experiences of sameness: "we are not like the others who make mistakes," and tolerate "destructive" experiences of difference: "we do not really belong." Unlike the destruction of the young child, the destruction of adolescence is substantially more pronounced and real. Hopefully, the groundwork of parents and their adolescence has been laid over time such that the destruction can occur without murder.

A note on the context of higher education

While we think that many adolescents are fully involved in these processes of becoming by the time they enter into college and universities, we also know that for whatever reason plenty are not. This means that there can be an interesting blend of students who are at different points in their consideration of self and other, which is part of both what gives higher education its appeal and can be a source of growing pains. Notably, higher education itself often positions on the side of facilitating destruction so to allow for elaboration of new ways of being.

This is especially true for liberal arts education. In these institutes, core classes and activities during orientation and onward are meant to challenge assumed knowledge about the world and comfortably held versions of being-ness in order to create the grounds for critical thinking, not just about ideas and topics but also, of course, about who one is. The role of the institute in these conversations is something we take up more fully in Chapter 7, but it is important to consider here the ways that adolescents bring the history of how they relate to authority and destruction into the new social and academic environments that college offers. As these legacies are complicated, we think it behooves our institutes to seriously consider how they engage students with these destructive and constructive processes.

While, historically speaking, the realm of relevance for this consideration is the classroom, we see increasingly that the institute as a whole, including the offices that administer athletic and residential programming, and psychological, career and academic counseling, must take on this role in grappling with how they relate to students. In this, we do not think that the institution has to serve as a "stand-in" or "replacement" for parents and caregivers. However, we *do* think that each institution must commit deliberately to consider how its own history and self-perception plays a role in facilitating or privileging certain emergent identities (and not others). This type of reflection is central to assessing the institution's overall success in meeting its educational mission.

Some examples of adolescence as a time for renewed destruction

There are, of course, plenty of reasons why an adolescent's wave may be prematurely collapsed as well as situations where the adolescent has been constrained from potentializing the dynamic of naming and un-naming in a wholesome way. As stated earlier, when the wave collapses into particular fixed points, identities or self-states, the self-system works to protect the self at the expense of further growth and development. This is when we expect the emergence of symptoms or difficulties in living. To a certain extent, this happens to all of us as we navigate the challenges of later childhood, adolescence, and early adulthood though sometimes the challenges are more extreme.

In her novel (1990, 1992), *Like Water for Chocolate*, Laurel Esquivel relates the terrible consequences of the collapse of potential being-ness. She does this, of course, in the way that only literature can capture so passionately and creatively.

Tita, the youngest daughter in a Mexican family, is bound by family tradition to forbear from exploration of herself as a sexual being who marries. Her role as an emerging adult is to devote herself entirely to the care of her aging mother. Her sexual being is limited to allowing Pedro, her sister's husband and her denied lover, to see her never-touched breasts in a moment of fleeting exposure while she grinds almonds for the meal she is preparing. Although in this moment her breasts embody an aspect of her sexual being-ness, this is something she cannot sustain. She is insistently subjugated to the will and desire of her mother, Elena, who scrupulously watches that no "fire" burn in or around Tita. Further, Tita can show no tears, sadness or signs of regret to others about her care-taking self-state. Her only recompense for her severely delimited life ("wave" of being) is that she had in his infancy suckled to health Pedro, her nephew (son of Pedro and her sister, Rosaura). However, on hearing that nephew, Pedro, has died, Tita's despair about the loss and her too singularly faceted life becomes overtly symptomatic. She devolves into muteness. She is then seen as *loca* (crazy) and taken away to Dr. John Brown's home for treatment.

Esquivel proceeds to convey succinctly what so often happens when someone like an adolescent immerses himself or herself into a context larger than that of the family. In the new context, there is opportunity, sometimes lifesaving, to redo and repair previous "collapses" of being-ness. Esquivel describes Tita's experience outside of the orbit of her mother as a freedom wherein she now felt she could do anything or become anything she desired. John, in his interactions with Tita, shares the wisdom of his grandmother which we, the authors, see as Esquivel's stunningly beautiful and sensual understanding about some aspects of the process of achieving object usage. Below we quote at length from Esquivel because no summary captures the resplendent elegance of her words:

> My grandmother ... said that each of is born with a box of matches inside ... but we can't strike them ... by ourselves; just as in an experiment, we need oxygen and the help of a candle to help. In this case the oxygen has to come, for example, would come from the breath of a person you love; the candle could be any kind of food, music, caress, word, or sound that engenders the explosion that lights one of the matches. Each person has to discover what will set off those explosions in order to live ... If one doesn't find out in time what will set off these explosions, the box of matches dampens, and not a single match will ever be lighted. (pp. 115–116)

Esquivel, however, goes on to say that John's grandmother warned that this lighting of the matches must be tempered. Lighting all the matches at once would produce "such a strong brilliance that before our eyes there would appear a tunnel of such radiance" that we would be called "back to our divine origins ... leaving the body lifeless" (1990, p. 117).

Here, Esquivel points almost poetically to the recognition that coming alive happens interpersonally, it happens in the process of interacting with an intimate other, and it happens with the oxygen from another that triggers a "fire" that lights the "matches" (the possibilities within us). The fire entails, of course, burning and therefore destruction, but it illuminates (being). It is also, however, a fire that must not be so great as to consume everything and thus lead to the death of being. It must, in other words, be a "lighting" that is "good enough" but does not ignore the limits of the "average ex-pectable environment." There must be oxygen from another that triggers the lighting of "one of the matches" (at a time or in measured time) but not so much oxygen (from another) that all possibilities for match-lightings are exhausted by one great, consuming conflagration.

Examples within universities and college contexts

We have frequently witnessed the dance of redoing or finding new being within the confines of our working with adolescents in uni-versity and college counseling centers. Although not the only place where this happens, college and universities are highly conducive to a second act, given their communitarian values and opportunities to live with peers and develop close almost parental relations with tea-chers, coaches, roommates and emerging friends. Of course, even with increased awareness afforded to marginalized and less re-presented students, some not only do not feel at "home" at their institute but also are in fact harmed by problematic structures and policies. While we take up these issues more extensively elsewhere (see, for instance, Chapters 7 and 8), it is necessary to keep this in mind.

Thus, while for many adolescence serves as a time of culturally sanctioned openness to looking beyond the culture of the family unit, it is rarely the idealistic process it is made out to be. As described above, it is precisely here that Ogden's interpretation of Winnicott makes sense. With openness comes destructive potential necessary to expand the wave. If circumstances are favorable, the adolescent en-counters others on their journey who help expand their potential zones of being so that previously unlit "matches" can light up and the wet wood of old matches dried sufficiently so that new "fire" can happen.

Notably, this process is not always easy. Shedding identities and moving into new skins can involve the destruction of previous iden-tities and with that the rejection of long-held compromises or at-tachments to other people's ideas or values. It may involve a renegotiation wherein multiple selves sit comfortably (or not) with each other, such that some are foregrounded in certain times and others at other times.

This is not without its own set of risks. Students sometimes report in "lighting" (enlightening) themselves, they set off multiple matches and then feel burnt out, overextended or at dangerous loose ends. At the authors' home college, there is a custom called "pluralism" where first years are organized by older students into groups for an extended evening of sharing. The lights are turned down low and a relaxed atmosphere is created. In this setting, students are encouraged to disclose one thing about themselves that other people there may not know. While this is a situation that many find to be an empowering opportunity for validation and greater intimacy, it is also not infrequently the case that a student in subsequent days will bemoan quite anxiously that they said "too much." "Lighting" is done in the bath of relating to others, but it must be done with an embracing and overarching understanding of how it is a dynamic and ongoing process.

Indeed, accessing the wave of one's being readily can meet obstacles and barriers. Creative growth and chaotic destruction may feel similar – both threatening. This was very much the case for Harry, a bi-racial, first generation, straight male for whom athletics held particular importance. Indeed, it was athletic issues that prompted him to access counseling and psychological services during his junior and senior years. A successful track athlete, Harry had long identified as a potential star in his sport. However, when he came to counseling, he was experiencing intense anxiety and depression. He reported drinking more heavily on the weekends, occasional forays into self-harm, and passive but present suicidal ideation.

In his appointments, it became apparent that much of his desire to run had originated with his father, a depressed controlling man who was not able to work and so was home almost all the time. Harry described how his father came alive during his races, vocally yelling encouragement and then spending days talking about Harry's form, speeds and expected competition. Harry felt trapped in his father's love of his athletic prowess. While he enjoyed racing, he did not enjoy the anxiety he felt before matches or the disappointment of his father when he ran poorly. In high school, this was compounded by the way dad could talk and disparage him after a bad race. No target was off-limit, including Harry's mother, whom dad felt was too "soft" on him. These attacks quickly strayed toward the abusive, and while Harry was never physically struck, on many occasions dad threw objects or flung emotional abuse.

Despite the clear sense that who Harry was had been collapsed into a singular construct for dad, Harry was incredibly reluctant to approach racing differently. Racing was the avenue for his attachment to dad, his prevailing intersect for receiving validating praise and reckoning with the glory and angry disappointment inherent to performance. Having internalized and identified with his father, Harry viewed other racers less dedicated than himself as weak or not committed.

Sessions felt like its own race between the therapist and Harry's self-destructive urges as it became increasingly understood that Harry held the wish to a "light a match" which both would illuminate newer possibilities for his own being-ness *and* the de-authorization of his father. This wish, of course, was held quite ambivalently, because Harry struggled to feel that embracing his own authority over that of his father's was not tantamount to dad's destruction as a person. Furthermore, Harry had internalized the authority of father to a great extent. For instance, even if dad was not at races where Harry performed poorly, he would tear into himself for being worthless. During these moments, he would drink alcohol often to a blackout point. Not surprisingly, his suicidality then would intensify. The therapist worried that in a fit of drunken rage, he'd seriously embody his destructive feelings.

In this capacity, the therapist struggled with how much to articulate his worry for him, fearful that he would be seen as the new controlling father who he had to live for. Eventually, the therapist articulated some of this worry, expressing both his desire to matter and offer hope but also his hope that Harry would not then experience him as the new sheriff to whose authority he had to validate and accede. In doing this, the therapist articulated what he thought was the part of Harry's self-system that wanted to give up running and pursue other things. This led to heated discussions about what "quitting" would mean and to the therapist inviting Harry to consider other views than his father's. Toward the end of junior year, Harry felt at last free enough to quit the track team. In asserting himself with father, he could say that it felt like dad's wishes, not his.

Harry was hoping to graduate and find a job that would allow him to not comply with dad's expectation that he return home. Senior year was filled with raising anticipation around job interviews, and he felt an anxiety reminiscent of what he felt before races. "What if I went into teaching? What if I became a lawyer? How about working for the government?" Each moment of possible growth was greeted by complicated internal "how could I?" judgments which Harry and his therapist had to explore respectfully before any new path actually could be pursued. In this way, Harry and his therapist weathered multiple storms that were fueled by his fear of disappointing his father and his desire to hurt father (exact painful retribution), all in the service Harry trying to find his own agentic wave.

By the time the treatment ended, Harry had found a job in a not-for-profit sector. While it lacked the trappings of success and competition longed for by himself and his father, the work felt meaningful and important to Harry. The therapist and Harry came to an agreement that Harry's working through his anxiety about being destructive allowed him a resolve that prompted dad's acceptance, even if begrudgingly, of Harry's post-college plan.

Summary

In this chapter, we engage Ogden's re-conceptualization of Winnicott, a re-consideration that entails insisting that mother must suffer a real destruction at the hand of their infant/child in order to facilitate a movement from object-relating to object usage. We argue that characterizing destruction as "real," while a useful step forward, maintains confusion about the infant's agency. Instead, we suggest a way of viewing development as a wave of potentiality, which can be collapsed at times but needs to also be expanded. From this perspective, real destruction is better suited for understanding the conduct of adolescents. We offer case examples to exemplify this.

Notes

1 This chapter is a version of a previous publication: Rosenbaum, P.J. & Webb, R.E. (2021). Appreciating Ogden's re-conceptualization of destruction but with a developmental arc: When is the big scary ape destructive? *Journal of Infant, Child, and Adolescent Psychotherapy.*

2 The words we put in quotes here are the ones commonly used by physicists. For readers largely unfamiliar with quantum physics they could read a short article (2015) by Chad Orzel titled, *Six Things Everyone Should Know About Physics.*

3 A wonderful example of this is found in Michael Cohen's book, Disloyal (2020). Cohen describes as a fifteen-year-old beginning to strut and talk "in 'dems and 'dos like a Brooklyn mobster" (p. 71), playacting this role so much that eventually his father confronted him and told him, "Cut it out … the whole mafia, gangster thing. You're not one of them" (p. 71).

References

Esquivel, L (1990). *Como agua para chocolate.* Planeta.

Esquivel, L (1992). *Like water for chocolate* (C Christensen, Trans.). Doubleday Books.

Hall, GS (1904). *Adolescence: Its psychology and its relation to physiology, anthropology, sociology, sex, crime, religion, and education* (Vols. 1 & 2). Prentice-Hall.

Klein, M (1975a). *The collected works of Melanie Klein, Volume I, love, guilt and reparation and other works 1921–1945.* The Free Press.

Klein, M (1975b). *The collected works of Melanie Klein, Volume III, envy, gratitude and other works 1946–1963.* The Free Press.

Lacan, J (1977). *Ecrits: A selection* (A Sheridan, Trans.).Norton. (Original work published 1966).

Lacan, J (1978). *The four fundamental concepts of psychoanalysis* (J Miller, Ed. & A Sheridan, Trans.). Norton. (Original work published 1956).

Ogden, T (1992a). The dialectically constituted/decentered subject of psycho-analysis. I. the Freudian subject. *International Journal of Psychoanalysis, 73* (3), 517–526.

Ogden, T (2016). Destruction reconceived: On Winnicott's 'The us of an object and relating through identifications'. *International Journal of Psychoanalysis, 97* (5), 1243–1262. 10.1111/1468-5922.5922.12341

Orzel, C (2015, July 8). Six things everyone should know about physics. *Forbes Magazine.* https://www.forbes.com/sites/chadorzel/2015/07/08/six-things-know-quantum-physics/#59a7d8017d46

Rosenbaum, PJ (2016). How self-harmers use the body as an interpretive canvas. *Culture & Psychology, 22* (1), 128–138. DOI: 10.1177/1354067X15 615814

Rosenbaum, PJ & Webb, RE (2021). Appreciating Ogden's re-conceptualization of destruction but with a developmental arc: When is the big scary ape destructive? *Journal of Infant, Child, and Adolescent Psychotherapy.* Advance online publication. 10.1080/15289168.2021.1879711

Rothman, J (2020, December 21). In another life, Making sense of who we might have been, *The New Yorker*, p. 69–73.

Winnicott, D (1969). The use of an object and relating through identifications. *International Journal of Psychoanalysis, 50*, 711–716.

Winnicott, DW (1971). *Playing and reality*. New York: Routledge Press.

Winnicott, D (1975). Hate in the countertransference. In *Through pediatrics to psycho-analysis* (pp. 194–203). Basic Books.

Zittoun, T, Duveen, G, Gillespie, A, Ivinson, G, & Psaltis, C (2003). The use of symbolic resources in developmental transitions. *Culture & Psychology, 9* (4), 415–448. 10.1177/1354067X0394006

Zittoun, T & Gillespie, A (2015). Internalization: How culture becomes mind. *Culture & Psychology, 21* (4), 477–491. 10.1177/1354067x15615809

Chapter 5

Developmental Considerations Associated with Suicide

Understanding and treating suicidal patients is among the most challenging and complex experiences that clinicians face, especially those working in university and college contexts. While being a student is considered a protective factor (Drum et al., 2009) and while the suicide rate for college students is significantly lower than the rate predicted for the general population (Schwartz, 2011), it remains a problem. According to the CDC (2009), approximately 1100 students make fatal attempts each year. This makes suicide the second leading cause of death of college-aged students. Along these lines, the American College Health Association's National College Health Assessment of Spring 2019 reports that more than 8% of students admit to thinking seriously about killing themselves. Similarly, Wilcox et al. (2010) found in their study that roughly 12% reported suicidal ideation during their four years with 2.6% reporting persistent ideation. Regardless of the specific data, there is no argument that suicide is a tragedy which because of its decision base has enhanced impact on us. Perhaps we might also say that there is something especially overwhelming about the suicide of a young person who has life at their feet.

Psychoanalysts, psychologists and suicidologists have helped clinicians and patients alike weather and work through suicidal states (Bateman & Fonagy, 2010; Maltsberger, 1998, 1993, 2004; Maltsberger & Buie, 1974, 1980; Tilman, 2016). They have explored and described how relationship triggers and vulnerabilities that seem to exist in the unconscious worlds of suicidal patients generate feelings of abandonment, loneliness, alienation and disconnection and how these feelings

DOI: 10.4324/9781003246558-6

can concretize thinking about the self and other, increase impulsivity, and ultimately lead to a collapse of self that results in such tremendous "psychache" (Shneidman, 1993) that suicide emerges as a significant possibility (Fowler, 2013; Goldblatt et al., 2018). From these perspectives, suicide is understood both as a way of ending pain and of expressing thoughts and feelings about intra- and interpersonal dilemmas that otherwise feel incommunicable.

The need for clinical theory in treating suicide in college and university settings

In this chapter, we offer clinical theory that pertains to understanding suicidal states that emerge at any age. We think, however, that having clinical theory to ground our efforts as therapists is especially important when we work in post-secondary institutional communities where we often have limited resources for intensive treatment and yet face the expectation that we assess and intervene with astute sensitivity and perspective. In contrast to an earlier era when sometimes students with "problems" where rather quickly hospitalized, sent home, or otherwise dismissed, presently, our greater sensibility about the civil rights of persons with psychological "disabilities" guides decision-making. It is now common for these students to be "held" within their college communities, often by teams at the counseling centers and other departments. Accordingly, we think that we as therapists who are at hand especially need ideas that help us locate ourselves and our patients in the challenge of finding life-sustaining relational connection when death to one of us might seem so resonant or inconsequential.

Moreover, as post-secondary institutions work to diversify their student population, increasing numbers of international students and those from less traditional backgrounds, the institution may find itself in the place of being, in effect, that student's home. So, while institutions still may assume only ambivalently comprehensive responsibility for their more vulnerable students, we think that providing robust care is an imperative that ethically proceeds from their concerted, marketing efforts. Since institutions often tout the diversity and the stimulating and caring qualities of their community as a reason for students to commit years of their life via enrollment, we view it as essential that the institution provide the actual resources (psychological, physical, spiritual and so forth) to make successful membership in the community a real possibility for all who are recruited.

Toward the end of hoping to add to the understanding of what so often can feel like an incommunicable dilemma about living, we focus in this chapter on suicide from a developmental perspective. We argue that in specific cases suicidal wishes and actions can be understood as emerging from impasses that limit the extent to which we are able to self-authorize and embrace agentic living. We specifically describe three configurations where functioning is impaired. The first two occur when we in some fundamental ways are not able to achieve a sense of agency or achieve it in a significantly compromised way. The third configuration addresses how we can lose grasp on our agency in the face of life's challenges, especially ones that so often emerge during late adolescence and young adulthood.

In keeping with our clinical thinking (Chapter 3), we note that it is our ability as therapists to form and sustain a relationship with our suicidal patient that is ultimately mutative. More about this we will discuss later, but for now, we note that we think our overall approach reflects what Mary Karr (1998) exhorts in her poem, *Incant Against Suicide* about not traveling into dark and scary places alone. We think that the creative application of theory can bring our patient's suicidal intentions into the relationship with us so that they do not travel there alone, especially when the theory helps us to fathom the phenomenological experience of patients as they try to negotiate the impasse in their developing sense of being-ness. That which frightens us (such as "spiders" for Karr) not only thwarts the patient's ability to engage life and living but also, of course, cast a defining shadow over the vitality of the therapeutic relationship.

The following statements we think aptly characterize the phenomenology of these impasses:

Configuration 1   *"I kill myself because I'm already dead."*
Configuration 2   *"I kill myself to prove that I'm alive."*
Configuration 3   *The thwarted embrace of our incompletion of being*:

   a   *"I kill myself to extinguish a profaned aspect of my being."*
   b   *"I kill myself to escape the intolerable chaos of new being."*
   c   *"I kill myself to proclaim the acceptance of me as I am that I do not receive in the recognition of others."*

Configuration 1: Restriction of being to the completion of "M-other" ("I kill myself because I'm already dead.")

The first developmental impasse arises out of our basic dependence upon our primary caregivers, the M-other. This dependence puts us at risk of becoming fixated on their will and desire. We encounter an impasse when our own uniqueness, our own no-thing-ness (Sartre, 1966) is elided in our relationship with M-other, preventing us from embodying meaningful experiences as a differentiated being (Benjamin, 1998). In other words, our burgeoning self is never allowed to articulate itself outside of the wishes and desires of the M-other and so our being-ness is not given space to truly come alive.

This occurs when the child's natural wish and need to ensure M-other's presence and availability joins with M-other's own anxiety about their essential incompleteness. In this case, the child serves as M-other's missing "phallus" (Lacan, 1966/1982). The potential for this enmeshment must be undermined through the availability and willingness of secondary caregivers (F-others) who support the aspects of M-othering that know that the child's destiny lies somewhere other than in being the M-other's ontological completion. In other words, "good enough" parents *together* exhort the child to look elsewhere for their life path, for their *partic*ularity from and within the whole-ness of their primary dependency. This involves the creative use of language to be able to name experiences in ways that are true to the child. From the perspective of Lacan (1977, 1993), the "name of the father" ("F-other") comes into play to represent the symbolic world outside the culture of the family home. Language (verbal and nonverbal, spoken and otherwise) is the means by which we both situate ourselves within the culture and by which we can construct new meaning to expand who we might become.

In Sullivan's appreciation of this "the interpretations of infancy, childhood and adolescence are of paramount concern. The transition from infancy to childhood is made possible by the learning of language and the organization of experience" (Lincourt & Olczak, 1974, p. 84). Learning language provides the child the freedom to symbolize and eventually to name themselves in a way that in the best progression entails full appreciation of Sartre's comment that *"[E]ssence* comes before *existence"* (1956/n.d., 7th paragraph, 3rd sentence, original emphasis).

When the primary caregiver restricts the child's language to being the extension of their desire, they, from the perspective of Sartre (1966), transform the child into an "in-itself" object rather than allowing the child to become a "for-itself" subject. Hence, as we noted earlier, the child cannot engage in new naming – a naming that would in some senses "un-name" – in the service of opening new ways of naming and, therefore, "being." They are, in other words, limited in their abilities to engage as semiotic beings who can partake in imaginative and constructive processes. In this situation, the potential anxiety that "naming/un-naming" entails threatens to shake the existential stability of the M-other, causing the child to remain stuck, unconsciously or not, in the deadness that adheres in fixated naming or objectification.

When this fundamental arrest happens, functioning is compromised in major ways, sometimes at a psychotic level, and almost always in a way that is accompanied by a sense of deep emptiness. When it does not overwhelm the person in despair, the emptiness is kept at arm's length by a retreat into a numbness of the person's "soul." When numbness prevails, staying alive as a breathing being is an onerous task that is meaningless because, whether breathing or not, they are already in spirit dead.[1]

Freud (1917) points our understanding in this direction. He says: "[T]he ego can kill itself only if ... it can treat itself as an object" (p. 252). Somewhat akin to this, Campbell (1999) writes about how it is the body of the suicidal person that becomes emblematic of objectification and, thereby, expendable. Underlining the dilemma of the person stuck with M-other without the intervention of F-other, Campbell says, "The good-enough father (sic) provides a model for identification as well as an alternative relationship to the child's regressive wish to return to a 'fusional' stay with mother (sic) with subsequent anxieties about engulfment" (p. 82).

Clinical implications and examples[2]

Sitting with these patients often entails tolerating what may feel to the therapist to be stifling, even maddening, deadness and disconnection. As befitting someone for whom language has never been allowed to become personally significant, there is scant foundation for expression, especially when it comes to trying to articulate something from within the internal world, the place where we experience our being to reside. As reflection of this, these patients usually demonstrate a severe restriction in their range of affect. Simultaneously, however, they somewhere within themselves experience an urgency to make connection which will allow them to spring more fully into living. The disconnections here create a difficult situation. The patient needs to be able to express themselves but also needs to learn how to do this. We think Francisco Gonzalez (2016) is addressing similar mental states when he writes:

> Working with primitive mental states ... can often mean waiting – and for long periods – without interpreting away the ruthless objectification of the person of the analyst. Questions of developmental arrest, of fixation, of basic fault, and environmental failure are all salient here. (p. 524)

Sustaining and developing a truly meaningful relationship with these patients often entails being able to manage long periods of silence and experiences of emptiness. In these periods, we, as therapists, are often considerably challenged to maintain our faith that we are *not* engaged in a futile effort.

Sometimes in the frustration of this, especially when therapy has space for extended and intensive work, we lose our hold on the "depth of despair and the experience of inner death" (McDougall, 1989, p. 93) that these patients embody, and we may in some way attack them, especially with our words. Joyce McDougall candidly reflects on her "ungraciously" (p. 93) referring to such patients as "the anti-analysand" (McDougall, 1972/1992). Nina Coltart reflects inspiringly about "an analyst's act of freedom as agent of change" (Symington, 1983/2017). She (Coltart, 2000) describes how in being "almost ... saturated in despair" by the utter silence of her patient, she "suddenly became furious and bawled [the patient] out for his prolonged lethal attack on [her] and on the analysis" (p. 10).

In short, it is a major challenge in the face of the inner deadness of these patients to bear in mind the phenomenology of their world ("I'm already dead") and the developmental impasse that makes their frequent resort to stifling silence an understandable reaction to having been so profoundly named by their primary caregiver. This can often appear like a power struggle between the therapist and patient, but this misses the feeling of powerlessness that the patient feels in trying to speak their experience. Speaking to these feeling, giving voice to the patients' experience of being with the analyst, of course, runs the risk of enactment (Levenson, 1983/2005), doing to the patient that which already has been done. However, not addressing it, may perpetuate the feeling of deadness on the patient and that no one will ever know and so give voice to their experience. It is here then that the analyst, may assume "the position of the law, of knowing and of authority, if only contingently, anxiously" (Gonzalez, 2016, p. 524).

In *not* speaking these patients seem to "speak" to the experience of having been so consumingly "spoken" for. They often gravitate to the "no-allowed-words-from-me" sanction they have suffered as a fledgling and unconscious way to demonstrate the slightest retribution available to them: "So if you want to do all the speaking, I'll leave you in full measure to do exactly that." Our challenge as therapists is to hear fully both elements of this dynamic so that we can better work to prevent the patient's despair from being so overwhelmingly encased within an experience of emptiness that suicide becomes the centralized option.

Alina was a heterosexual, cis-gender female international first-year student who presented to the college counseling center shortly after arriving on campus hoping to make a connection with a therapist in order to meet with a psychiatrist and continue to receive medications (as per the policy of the center). She sat in silence during the session, providing short monotone answers to the questions about the reasons for wanting medication. She described depression and anxiety but without any details. Her relationships were "fine," "okay" and "good." Due to limited financial means, she felt unable to see an off-campus psychiatrist. Despite the relative silence, the therapist felt some small connection, as did Alina, so they agreed to meet weekly.

During her first semester, Alina was dominated by the silencing of her objectified naming. Alina would come in, sit, often not taking off her coat, and wait to be asked questions. Her answers were sparse and short. She did not provide details about her interpersonal world, her inner world, her transition to college, her experiences prior, her family and so forth. However, she also rarely missed appointments, and the silence did not feel hostile. Instead, there was a pensiveness about her, a searching and almost yearning feeling the therapist could later understand as perhaps reflecting her hope for naming which could "un-name" her.

At points, the therapist tried to language the silence, remarking to her about how it felt to him: that it were as if she did not have words to speak or sufficient hope that speaking *her* words would really matter. Other times, he would speak about his thoughts and feelings about the silence, noting especially how heavy it felt.

Right before the end of the first semester, when acknowledging the coming winter break, Alina indicated that she would miss having the sessions. This seemed to indicate that the therapist's efforts were more meaningful to her than her relative silence might suggest, and so it augured well for the possibility of the work being able to progress following the break-instituted separation. When she returned, although she was still more silent than not, she was sometimes able to punctuate her presence with stories about home. A picture of intrusive grandparents emerged. Both her parents were busy working in a different part of her country, and she was raised by her mom's parents. In this special, necessary arrangement, she was expected to do her part; she was expected to be minimally needy and to demonstrate this by succeeding in an effortless and unobtrusive fashion.

Her grandmother eventually emerged as someone who Alina experienced as having virtually no psychological space to embrace her complexities as an emerging woman. Grandmother, instead, seemed only to be able to center herself on how Alina's always smooth and successful interaction with the world was a rock upon which Grandmother reliably could rest her pride. An Alina without problems made her a special caregiver. Eventually, many stories came into words to exemplify this, but one was particularly emblematic of it to Alina. She recalled the awful experience of being teased by peers about her menarche. When she got home and asked for help, grandmother skipped past the depth of this request and concretized it as a simple inquiry about hygiene care, thus a matter that with but brief instruction Alina as a "good girl" could surely and quietly address by herself.

Not surprisingly, suicidal fantasies frequented Alina's imagination. In almost all versions of these killing of herself, she imagined taking just enough prescribed medication so that she would go to sleep and never wake up. In eventually being able to speak of this in a more elaborated way, she maintained that her death would be inconsequential. It was clearly evident that since she felt so empty of distinct being-ness, it eluded her expectation that she would be truly missed as a person. Only very slowly over the course of considerable work with her college therapist did this suicide wish transform into a wish that she could sleep and wake up, but wake up as some metamorphosed version of herself.

Configuration 2: Collapse of being into the completion of "F-other" ("I kill myself to prove that I'm alive.")

Our second interpersonal configuration picks up where the first leaves off. Recall that the F-other, ideally with the support of the M-other, introduces the child to culture and language to facilitate a movement outside of the initial M-other child continuity and completion. Lacan, working with the hegemony of Freud's concepts but seeking to also differentiate himself from them, refers to this as the F-other's role in "castrating" the "phallus" role (Lacan, 1966/1982). Again, we emphasize that we need not sex this F-other role with a "father." Instead, we are speaking of a relational function by which a caregiving authority communicates to the child that the orbit of their life needs to go beyond their primary attachment and *also* beyond the delimiting orbit of the F-other authority who insists on this. In other words, the F-other must not replace the M-other in asserting that the child lives as a completion for an-other. The child's worthiness is embraced and sustained by their knowing that the destiny for their being-ness is their own; it is not destiny found by pursuing someone else's (Chapter 1).

Failure in this F-other role not only returns the child to being the articulation of someone else's desire but is also a dangerous "bait and switch." The child is first told that their destiny is not M-other's and then told that they are to be someone else's completion. This subverts the child's burgeoning agency and subjectivity as well as their necessary confrontation with our essential, existential aloneness in the world, an understanding that entails both the overwhelming and joyful realization that we can participate in naming themselves.

When F-other replaces M-other in using the child as a narcissistic extension of their own needs and desires, they are insisting upon an untenable idealization of themselves as the new object of completion. In the parlance of Lacan, the developmental play that is at hand is that the

> father (sic) does not make the child the object of his desire and is not the desire of the child" [but understands and communicates that] he does not have the phallus as the satisfaction of desires but as a symbol. (Webb et al., 1997, p. 9)

What makes obstruction in this process especially insidious is that the child has been introduced into a culture and language, but one with which they then cannot participate on their own terms. In some sense, we might say that the child has been shown the possibility of greater being only to be barred from participation in it.

We see the suicidal condition that emerges in this situation as similar yet significantly different from our first position. Recall that the child in the first position has never truly been allowed to be alive and so feels empty. However, in this next position, F-other is bigger than life, and the despair of not having access to meaningful participation in naming oneself is now contained not so much by emptiness but by rage. Whereas in the first position the child is transformed into an object "in itself," in the second they taste the freedom of being a subject "for themselves" only to then be forced back into the role of an object.

Here, rage is much more prominent, the impassioned anger at having been deprived the opportunity they had experienced, even if only in a glimpsing way. This rage then is expressed with words like "I refuse" and "I absolutely will not," and can erupt with an existential urgency that befits the high stakes at play (but which is also within the same ballpark of meaning as the toddler child who, in their nascent sense of personhood, must with "no" define themself as separate before the "yes" that reflects convergence with another can be accommodated. In some important ways, "no" must precede "yes"). When the position of "I will not" emerges, it must be acknowledged within an appreciation of the emptiness and terror of not-being that lies behind it.

Clinical implications and examples

From within this position, the potential for seeking death is more actively embraced and thus its suicidal nature is much less ambiguous. If we characterize the first position's suicidal feeling as a persistent drone, in the second position the feeling is more a tonal note which flashes into fortissimo play. In other words, in contrast to the first configuration the rage of the individual and the need to refuse can fuel actions that in their surge can be harder to anticipate than the vacuous depression that is so consuming and ever-present in the first position. The feelings of rage at the bait and switch and the experience of having our burgeoning agency cut off generate intense affect. Accordingly, sustaining a relationship with a patient is different here than with the first configuration, which requires our being at peace with sitting with inchoate subjectivity. Here, we have to survive the patient's intense affective states in order to understand and even experience them. This means not only observing and being curious but sometimes tolerating and living through dramatic actions of a patient's "refusals to live." We hasten to remind the reader that patients can move between the configurations. In fact, treatment progress requires such movement. Hence, we make note of the rather common observation that suicide often comes when the "depression" is lifting, and we proffer that this can reflect the movement from the first to the second configuration.

Within the college counseling context, these "refusals to live" often reflect what can be the bewildering situation of living in a space with the expressed intent of exploring and experiencing one's agency but without the conviction that this is possible. This was the case for Sam, a cis-gendered Caucasian, first-year student from a politically conservative family. Sam had grown up in his father's shadow. Dad was in many ways larger than life. He was deeply involved in local politics, and his questioning of the validity of vaccines and endorsement of various conspiracy theories was proclaimed loudly and passionately both within the family and in the community. He insistently warned Sam about "radical liberals" on campus who would attempt to "convert" him, and he implored Sam to stand up for the conservative truths that had nurtured him. Sam was sunk in feeling himself authorized to represent dad but not to explore his own interests and viewpoints. In a sense, he was a secret agent meant to fight the life around him but not to partake of it. His mandate was to be a placeholder for F-other but not a subject "for-itself" (Sartre, 1966).

The weight of this burden, of course, fell hard and swiftly on Sam as his natural desire to make a home for himself within his new community at college surged within him. If only in a partially conscious way, Sam longed to immerse himself as a *free agent* in both the social and intellectual life of the college. Of course, Sam had little foundation for embracing this agency; being himself, whatever that might be, was fraught. His dilemma became more acutely experienced when his sexuality stirred in ways which placed him clearly outside of dad's sanctioned possibilities for being-ness. As the semester proceeded the tension built. Sam would spend a weekend partying and hooking up with "guys and girls" and then be awash in guilt which exacted punishment through social retreat. In his isolation, he would not do his schoolwork but instead spend hours zoning out on the internet, sporadically but also both dreadfully and excitedly looking for "authoritative" posts and websites about bi-sexuality.

Sam continually faltered in his effort to communicate to his dad his own sense of self-discovery. Sam could not tolerate seeing dad upset or disappointed, and so he pretended to him that he was keeping with the "mission." Simultaneously, he could not connect with other people about his struggles. While some may have suspected that his excessive lifestyle tilted from inner struggle, he kept his confusion and conflicts to himself. Things reached a boiling point around the political activities of the fall, where in the throes of "watch" parties and debates Sam "lost it." He smashed his computer through his dorm room window. When caring hall mates came running to investigate, he dissolved into an explosion of tears and exclaimed his wish to jump to his death. An upper-class "head resident" shared with Sam his own trust of talking to someone at CAPS, and Sam acceded in a relieved way to this possibility of "new authority." He met with a therapist on an emergency basis and entered into the treatment which revealed the story noted earlier.

Configuration 3: The thwarted embrace of our incompletion of being

We think this third configuration can be exemplified by several phenomenological positions that can emerge once we have embodied a significant sense of our agency within the naming/un-naming dynamic of being-ness. This impasse results from what are sometimes thought of as narcissistic wounds or injuries. Whether we are afflicted by our own actions or that of an other, we face an undigestible challenge to our sense of who we are or have imagined ourselves to be. As a result, we lose the dynamic nature of our being, and we feel overwhelmingly stuck within a state that defines us. Unbearable shame and feelings about our "badness" predominate. From this perspective, we cannot imagine moving past this emphatically evident iteration of our being. We feel that "There is no way back" and so suicide seems to be the only way forward.

Notably, the challenges described here are in many ways typical of the challenges of living. They are the ordinary setbacks, mistakes, and experiences which we are all susceptible to making and feeling; the times when we hurt someone, make a grievous error, or act irresponsibly (see William Butler Yeats' (1962/1932) poem, *Vacillation*, for the beautifully captured expression of this). On the surface, while humiliating and humbling, it is not clear that these events in "being" should precipitate a suicidal crisis, and yet they sometimes do. We must never gainsay the possible distance in meaning between what is manifest and that which is subtextual.

What precipitates seeing suicide as a solution to these problems we locate within the developmental processes that entail de-authorization of our caregivers. Recall that our caregivers have to allow us the existential space to experience our abilities to name and un-name ourselves. To do this they must introduce us to culture and then cede to our own desire to express the truths that are personally meaningful to us. In step with this, they must accept themselves as flawed beings who hold no privileged authority about Truth. By doing this, they support our looking for our own subjectivity both within our relationship with them and outside of our relationship to them (Chapter 1).

When this process is successful, our caregivers serve to relativize culture and language. It allows not only for the de-authorization of themselves as the final arbitrator of right and wrong but sets the ground for contextualizing all societal constructs ("big F-other") that guide meaning-making, such as in religion and politics. Within this context of dismantled authority, we come to learn that there are no external forces, such as "the church," a "favored philosopher/teacher" or a "political party" that have and can hold all the answers.

This emergent understanding introduces the stark and painful existential fact that we ultimately have both the exciting and the suffering responsibility in life for articulating within ourselves what is good and ethical. Per Sartre (1956/n.d.),

> When a man commits himself to anything, fully realizing that is not only choosing what he will be, but is thereby at the same time a legislator deciding for the whole of mankind – in such a moment a man cannot escape from the sense of complete and profound responsibility. (paragraph 11, lines 2–4).

When, for whatever reason, we are not able to recognize the relativity of our experience and that there is no final arbitrator of truth, we render ourselves susceptible to narcissistic injuries and wounds that can leave us profoundly shaken. We lose conviction that we can re-engage our sense of self through new naming. Instead, we feel profound shame, anger, and upset about the *who we are* that we have foreclosed upon. From here, suicide can emerge to us as a reasonable choice.

In what follows we describe three iterations of how this might appear. These are as follows:

a   With suicide, we might seek to cleanse our self with self-destructive judgment ("I will kill myself to extinguish a profaned aspect of my being").

b   Suicide might seem to us to be a permanent escape from the turmoil that accompanies the challenge of assimilation and accommodation ("I will kill myself to escape the intolerable chaos of being").

c   Suicide provides a manic (Winnicott, 1975) search for recognition and to get in the last word ("I will kill myself to proclaim my acceptance of me").

A   *"I will kill myself to extinguish a profaned aspect of my being"*

For college students, this first position entails considerable risk. Having not had as much experience in living as older adults, there is greater possibility that they will encounter academic, career or social setbacks with the tremendous shame and despair that often comes with the rawness of new encounters. Notably, we think that these experiences need to be grappled with and understood by us as therapists with as close alignment as possible with these students' phenomenological and lived experiences. We proffer that labeling adolescents in these situations as "fragile" or "lacking resilience" alienates both student and adult from each other and can reflect the anxiety of broader culture about recognizing the semiotic grounds within which students are coming into their agency as meaning-makers. Indeed, with so much effort being put into the professionalization of college students there is an increasing sense that what happens during the college years is essentially a life or death matter.

Hence, it is *not* moralizing which is helpful here but rather heartfelt interest in looking at what is so grievously at play that the student's sense of being feels "profaned." Certainly, this was the case for Miguel a first-generation college student from an immigrant family. Cis-gendered and heterosexual, Miguel suffered from a learning disability which at the time of his seeking help was still undiagnosed. Like so many other students do, he had compensated through his natural brilliance during high school but then come to college with anxiety and dread that he would be "found out" as a "fraud."

As if both to compensate but to make this true, he took a demanding course of study his first semester and performed poorly. Facing the deep fear of what he thought this achievement "slip" revealed about his true self and the shame of disappointing his family, Miguel began seriously to contemplate suicide. The expectations that his success would "lift the family up" were crushing him with both pride and fear. His musings fueled late-night walks about campus and sometimes uncontrollable sobbing sessions on a bench a bit off the main trail. The happenstance of an engaged conversation with a campus safety officer during one of these episodes is what fostered his coming to the counseling service.

B   *"I will kill myself to escape the intolerable chaos of being"*
Sometimes during our work with college students, suicide emerges at points that may from the outside seem surprising. This can be when students are in meaningful therapeutic relationships but looking for

ways of being which offer promise of better representing how they experience themselves. However, when we look more closely, what we sometimes find is that these students are on the edge. Although they need to and even want to embrace newer way of being, such embrace comes with great hesitation. Moving beyond accustomed ways of being generates the fear of losing important relationships and living with the chaos of "not knowing" that inhabits change. If the disordered process that precedes growth is too overwhelming, then the possibility of suicide enters into the picture.

Sammy, a single bi-sexual cis-gender senior female presented to the counseling center feeling overwhelmingly confused, depressed and anxious. For her senior thesis in religion, she was writing about the eschatology of a variety of German, existential theologians. As she dived deeply into what she understood to be the fundamental demand of original Christianity for embodying agape, she simultaneously involved herself in political protests against US policies that were separating immigrant children from their parents. During spring break, she arranged to immerse herself in work at an agency on the southern border of the country that offered food and legal counsel to immigrants living in make-do tent "cities."

Sammy connected deeply with a young mother who shared with Sammy her consuming fear of returning to her home country but also her fear that her children would be separated from her if she pushed forward with her efforts to find sanctuary in the United States. When Sammy's week-long break from college was coming to a close, she had a heart-wrenching goodbye with this peer of drastically different circumstance. Now back within the safe confines of the college community, Sammy could hardly bear to eat without blistering herself with condemnation for not following the demands of what she now understood to be true Christian love. She dwelled on the serendipity of life that assigned her secure life. She viewed her return to the college as a devastating indictment of her failure in courage to live the principles that she said that she believed in and which she thought would require her to abandon her studies and take meaningful and immediate action to make the world better. Reassurances from friends and family with whom she shared her angst were experienced as efforts to mollify her. In her despair about the hypocrisy of others, and, most importantly herself, she drank herself into oblivion on a street in a high crime area of the city and hoped to be fatally assaulted. A charity outreach worker found her shivering in an alley among homeless clients and alerted the police who contacted college officials who eventually got her to agree to see a CAPS counselor.

C *"I will kill myself to proclaim the acceptance of me as I am that I do not receive in the recognition of others"*

Our final example speaks to the collapse of self that comes when we feel unrecognized or unseen by the world, even sometimes by our own family. Then, in a manic search for recognition suicide becomes an option of proclaiming the injustice of our situation and of affirming our very being. Not surprisingly, this often can be the case for college students whose history of being unseen may lead to fantasies about being noticed during their college years. When they are not noticed or when they realize that they will have to work in order to make relationships, they can be filled with resentful rage and anger and so look toward suicide as a way of expressing their powerful array of feelings.

Jamie, a heterosexual, cis-gender black college sophomore, had spent most of his life in the shadow of his younger brother. His brother was a high achieving student, athletically talented, and socially popular. He was the family's future doctor. Jamie, on the other hand, was middle-of-the-road in everything. While he got passable grades in his academic work, graduate work and a career as a multiply degreed professional was neither likely or to his liking. He voiced no ambitions that his family thrilled about. While he had a few significant friends, he thought most peers viewed him as the big boy edition of the clumsy kid that everyone picked on in middle school. In fact, Jamie had learned to use being a scapegoat in really adaptive ways by turning his perceived foolery into endearing farce. Occasionally, he had opportunity to do this on campus, but at home with his family he experienced himself as more talked past than talked to. In other words, within the family, he felt he was a quiet unknown, who could generate little curiosity about himself. He thought that his being ignored should be viewed as generous kindness that stood in place of disappointment-fueled prodding. In short, he had little opportunity to float into open what he thought might be his comedic talent.

However, once at college Jamie began slowly but progressively to explore the nearby city's community of comics. He first started simply going to shows, occasionally with a friend but just as often by himself. As time proceeded some of the comics began to recognize him in the audience. "One thing led to another," and soon Jamie was doing open mike night on a regular basis. He got good, and as he gained a local reputation as up and coming, he looked with eager anticipation to a special show where a male and female comic from among the collective of performers would be chosen by the audience for a sizable cash award.

Jamie took the plunge. Not only did he register himself to perform but also invited his parents to attend. They said they would "try," but noted that his brother had a basketball game that night. They didn't show. In retrospect, Jamie saw that he didn't entirely contextualize for his parents how important their coming was to him, but he also verbalized to his therapist that he's asking them to attend any activity of his that entailed his active involvement was unprecedented. "Why couldn't they see that? Why couldn't they divine how important this was to me?"

Jamie won, and he went back to his dorm room and cut his wrists. The next day when the parents came to the hospital, they had in hand the note he left them with the award check signed over to them.

Clinical positioning: "Don't go there alone"

From our perspective, thinking about developmental impasses that may lead to suicidal crises and actions helps to inform how we situate ourselves clinically with patients. We try to keep in heart and mind our patient's existential-relational positions and the related impasses as an ongoing way of asking ourselves where our patient and where we are in relationship to each other and the life that surrounds us. In this regard, the configurations help us think about the role(s) the patient may be asking us to play within the transference-countertransference interactions. Moreover, these configurations help us understand and tolerate the patient's conscious and unconscious feeling states, including intense levels of despair, suffering and pain, as well as anger and hate.

What is then foundational for working with suicidal patients is conveying in more than just words our commitment to being with them, to being in relationship with them, among all their (and our) feelings about living and dying. With respect to this, some variation of the following is something in one way or another, we especially find ourselves communicating to our patients in the first two configurations:

> If you are going to kill yourself, which I most dearly hope you won't ultimately feel you must do, I want you to do so in the context of your relationship to me. Towards the end of trying to live, we must somehow find a bridge to the world of words.

To embody the above position, we certainly must seek to be steady. This is something that Mashud Khan[3] helps us with when he says: "In our clinical work, sometimes, it is more important to sustain a person in living than to rid him of his illness" (Khan, 1983, p. 97). Khan made this statement in appreciation of Donald Winnicott's comment that "... absence of psycho-neurotic illness may be health, but it is not life" (1971, p. 100). Khan and Winnicott allude here to the idea that being without symptom, whether that is suicidality, depression, anger, or whatever, does not mean that the patient is alive. Referring to Winnicott's statement, Khan says: "If we try to subvert his [the patient's] life by a cure, he either escapes us or gives up his right to be alive and ill and enters into a complicity with us that we mistake for 'treatment alliance'" (1983, p. 97).

In other words, if our patient experiences our priority to be their cure rather than an appreciation and understanding of their attempt at living, as expressed through their suicidality, we risk substituting ourselves for the other from whom the patient is already struggling to differentiate themselves. We may in fact become a new version of this demanding other and reenact the impasse with them in a collusive way. The anxiety, fear, and hate that suicide can arouse puts us at risk of engaging our own incompletion and anxieties as a therapist in such a way that we insist the patient give up their symptom, the unfathomed meaning of their suicidality, in a false compliance of living for us. This can come from even well-intentioned efforts by analysts to name the patient's unconscious fantasies, conflicts and wishes, preoccupying their efforts with theories and techniques that emphasize "knowing" and "interpretation," rather than sitting in the muddy waters that the uncertainty of relating entails, risk this dangerous substitution.

Being attuned to the relational configuration at play is not, then, a simple matter of applying a template in pursuit of a solution. Instead, it is having an idea of the impasse a patient may be stuck within and offering them, as Kahn says, "concrete space to be in and ... [also] potential space where they [can] sustain moods and larval psychic experiences that their ego-capacities cannot yet actualize" (1983, p. 99). In short, our task is to be where our patient is and, within this, both to provide and create the space for potential for new forms of being. Using a title of one of Winnicott's books as an evocative way of capturing this, we might say "home is where we start from" (1986).

Toward this end, it would probably be simpler for therapists if the relatively discrete categories we described mapped singularly onto the situations of our suicidal patients or if their plight could be understood from a metapsychological perspective. However, as stated earlier, the manifestations of these impasses typically do not fit neatly into the frames that our clinical examples suggest. The truth is that there is usually a layered fluid complexity in the manifestation of these impasses. However, listening with an ear toward the relationship(s) that a patient is struggling with can inform how we sit with that patient as they try to move toward living.

Hearing that a patient is stuck in the despair of having never truly lived because of trying to live for their caregiver is and feels different than someone who feels stuck after having tasted the freedom of being their own person only then to be collapsed. Still more complicated are the half measures by which a patient might have achieved some independence but remain partially stuck. So also, are the situations by which the patient has learned that they can never truly be enough and so feel that nothing they do will amount to anything.

To sustain a person in living is without doubt complicated and demanding. We suggest that it involves appreciating a dual-leveled meaning of a phrase coined by Erna Furman. She, although speaking of parents, says something which we think apt for understanding our role as therapist. We must "be there to be left" (1982, p. 15).

At *one* layer of meaning, this involves allowing ourselves to be a real other with the patient. While we agree that the patient must ultimately come to life on their own terms, we also must allow them to experience within the relationship our desire to experience them as a being who is actively considering dying. To truly be left we and the patient have to be present in an ongoing way, a demand that at times can require heartfelt caring. An entreaty that the patient stays within the relationship and within the world of words rather than move into life-ending action. The patient needs to feel that their inclusion and continuity in the whole is important.

"To be there to be left" has also another layer of meaning that is essential to hold in concert with the first. Here, we hope that the relationship can embrace the paradox that we, as therapists, are saying "Stay here so that I can be left on terms of you coming to life." In this stance, we are working ultimately to support a "being left" which entails our de-authorization and the patient's self-authorization. This is a movement which begins when the patient is able to use the relationship we have with them as the potential space that Kahn notes earlier, the space to find new experiences at being.

We hasten to note that being a real other with whom a suicidal patient fathoms questions about "Why should I live?" is a tricky and harrowing business. In "the home from which we start" there is almost always "What difference is there between living for you and living for my mother or father?" and/or "Prove to me that I am not an abomination, not worth the shit that I expel?" In trying to matter enough to the patient that they can experience conflict around desire and being without imposing other stagnating demands upon them, we walk at times the narrowest and most slippery of tightropes. If we fail to bring new hope but rather dead air, we can precipitate a new suicidal crisis.

We add that once suicide is considered within the relationship, we do not rule out an intervention that embodies the statement:

> I am holding for you a wish for life that you cannot feel right now. You might hate me right now for insisting that you be in a safe place (e.g., a hospital). I'm hoping one day soon you'll understand that I am doing what I do, because I care that you have time to find your aliveness, and I take seriously the struggles you have been sharing with me.

For instance, patients who are in the throes of raging at their caregiver's inability to relativize themselves and who are full of destructive rage may impulsively turn to self-destruction as a means of expressing their self-articulation to an-other (F-other) who almost certainly will not hear. In these cases, we must hear the rage and with it the impulsivity toward self-harm as a wish to annihilate, to separate from being the will of F-other (and also perhaps the therapist). So, it might only be through a hospitalization that the crisis of rage can pass sufficiently that the patient can get in touch with more helpless and despairing feelings. Similarly, with patients who have suffered severe narcissistic wounds, as we have described earlier, we might hear their desire to kill off the bad identity. However, we might act in a way to protect the rest of the self so that living can resume more fully.

Moreover, in acting within the relationship (a hospitalization) even as the patient moves to enact outside of it, we present ourselves as a potentially new caregiver (parent, mother, father, or societal other) with whom the client can struggle. While this in fact might lead to discussions about living and dying (and we can even imagine acting) we think it does so within the confines of a therapeutic relationship. Notably, if we fail to embrace our own existential anxiety about choice and not knowing, we run the risk of appearing to the patient as inauthentic and not grappling seriously with their crisis.

What is needed is not an insistence upon cure but rather space for sustaining a relationship of exploration and curiosity which invites new possibilities for being. With this curiosity also comes a willingness to engage with all of our patients' selves, even those that live in dark corners. It is for this exploration that we encourage steadiness and perseverance.

Summary

In this chapter, we describe how suicide can be understood differently depending upon where and how we situate our patients' developmental impasses. We described what we think happens during these developmental impasses that we think lead patients to consider suicide as an option and help us approach creating and sustaining relationships with them. While suicidal thoughts, feelings and actions are multifaceted and so do not fit neatly into these categories we hope to have demonstrated how considering patients' existential-relational positioning helps inform our own clinical posturing.

Notes

1 For readers disposed toward how literature offers us expression of our complex human condition, Laura Esquivel captures the essence of this numbed despair in her character, Tita, in her novel, *Like Water for Chocolate* (1990, 1992).
2 In our article noted above which is under editorial review we offer a case which reflects intensive treatment over many years and which delves into transference and countertransference issues in an in- depth way. In this chapter, we try to restrict ourselves to case material that pertains more directly to our work with students.
3 We realize that Khan is a very controversial figure. Our referencing some of his published ideas is not an endorsement of reports of how he conducted himself as either a person or analyst. Sometimes worthy truth is spoken not only out of the mouth of babes but from any person regardless of how personally they live their life.

References

ACHANCHA II, American College Health Association National College Health Assessment, Spring 2019, Reference group data Report, https://www.acha.org/documents/ncha/NCHA-II_SPRING_2019_US_REFERENCE_GROUP_DATA_REPORT.pdf accessed Feb 22, 2021.

Bateman, A & Fonagy, P (2010). Mentalization based treatment for borderline personality disorder. *World Psychiatry: Official Journal of the World Psychiatric Association (WPA)*, 9 (1), 110–115. 10.1002/j.2051-5545.2010.tb00255.x

Benjamin, J (1998). *Like subjects love objects: Essays on recognition and sexual difference.* Yale University Press.

Campbell, D (1999). The role of the father in a pre-suicide state. In RJ Perelberg (Ed.) *Psychoanalytic understanding of violence and suicide* (pp. 75–86). Routledge.

Centers for Disease Control and Prevention. (2009) *Web-based Injury Statistics Query and Reporting System (WISQARS) [online]* National Center for Injury Prevention and Control; Atlanta. [Google Scholar].

Coltart, N. (2000). *Slouching towards Bethlehem.* Other Press.

Drum, DJ, Brownson, C, Denmark, AB & Smith, SE (2009). New data on the nature of suicidal crises in college students: Shifting the paradigm. *Professional Psychology*, 40 (3), 213–222. 10.1037/a0014465

Esquivel, L (1992). *Like water for chocolate* (C Christensen, Trans.). Doubleday Books, 1992.

Fowler, JC (2013). Core principles in treating suicidal patients. *Psychotherapy, 50* (3), 268–272. 10.1037/a0032030.

Freud, S (1917). Mourning and melancholia, *Standard Edition, 14*, 237–260.

Furman, E (1982)/ Mothers have to be there to be left. *The Psychoanalytic Study of the Child, 11* (1), 15–28. 10.1080/00797308.1 982.11823356

Goldblatt MJ, Herbstman, B, Schechter, M, Ronningstam, E (2018). John Terry Maltsberger, American psychoanalyst: Contributions to the development of studies of suicide and self-attack. *Journal of the American Psychoanalytic Association, 66* (5), 861–882. 10.1177/0003 065118801596.

Gonzalez, F (2016). On the relation to non-relationality. *Psychoanalytic Dialogues, 26* (5), 522–531. 10.1080/10481889909539308

Karr, M (1998). *Viper rum*. New Directions.

Khan, M (1983). *Hidden selves, Between theory and practice in psycho-analysis*. Maresfield Library.

Lacan, J (1977). *Ecrits: A selection* (A Sheridan, Trans.). W.W. Norton. (Original work published 1966).

Lacan, J (1982). The meaning of the phallus. In J.Mitchell & J Rose (Eds.), *Feminine sexuality, Jacques Lacan and the école Freudienne* (pp. 74–85). Norton. (Original work published 1966).

Lacan, J (1993). *The psychoses, The seminar of Jacques Lacan. Book III 1955-1956* (J-A Miller, Ed. & R Grigg, Trans.). Routledge.

Levenson, EA (1983/2005). *The Ambiguity of Change*. Routledge Press.

Lincourt, JM & Olczak, PV (1974). C.S. Peirce and H.S. Sullivan on the human self. *Psychiatry, 37*, 78–84. 10.1080/00332747.1974.11023789

Maltsberger, J (1993). Confusion of the body, the self, and others in suicidal states. In *Suicidology: Essays in Honor of Edwin S. Shneidman* (pp. 148–171). Aronson.

Maltsberger, JT (1998). Suicide danger: Clinical suicide danger: Clinical estimation and decision. *Suicide & Life-Threatening Behavior, 18* (1), 47–54. 10/1111/j/1943-278x.1988.tb00140.x

Maltsberger, J (2004). The descent into suicide. *International Journal of Psychoanalysis, 85* (3), 653–667. 10.11516/3c96-uret-tlwx-6lwu

Maltsberger, J & Buie, DH (1974). Countertransference hate in the treatment of suicidal patients. *Archives of General Psychiatry, 30* (5), 625–633. 10.1001/archpsyc.1974.01760110049005

Maltsberger, JG & Buie, DH (1980). The devices of suicide: Revenge, riddance, and rebirth. *International Review of Psycho-Analysis, 7* (1), 61–72.

McDougall, J (1989). *Theaters of the body, A psychoanalytic approach to psychosomatic illness.* W.W. Norton.

McDougall, J (1992). *Plea for a measure of abnormality.* Brunner/Mazel. (Original work published 1972).

Sartre, J (n.d.). *Existentialism as humanism.* https://www.marxists.org/reference/archive/sartre/works/exist/sartre.htm (Original work published 1956).

Sartre, J-P (1966). *Being and nothingness, a phenomenological essay on ontology* (HE Barnes, Trans.) Washington Square Press. (Original work published 1943).

Shneidman, ES (1993). *Suicide as psychache: A clinical approach to self-destructive behavior.* Jason Aronson.

Schneiderman, S (1990). Art as symptom: A psychoanalytic study of art. In PC Hogan & L Pandit (Eds.), *Criticism and Lacan on Language, Structure, and the Unconscious* (pp. 207–222). Univ. of Georgia Press.

Schwartz, AJ (August 01, 2011). Rate, Relative Risk, and Method of Suicide by Students at 4-Year Colleges and Universities in the United States, 2004-2005 through 2008- 2009. *Suicide and Life-Threatening Behavior, 41* (4), 353–371. 10.1111/j.1943-278X.2011.00034.x

Symington, N (2017). *The analyst's act of freedoms as agent of therapeutic change.* Routledge. 10.4324/9781351262880-16 (Original work published 1983).

Tilman, JG (2016). The intergenerational transmission of suicide: Moral injury and the mysterious object in the work of Walter Percy. *Journal of the American Psychoanalytic Association, 64* (3), 541–567. 10.1177/0003 065116653362

Webb, RE, Bushnell, DF, & Widseth, JC (1997). The birth and death of desire: the Significance of Lacan's "Name of the Father" in work with the sexually abused. *Clinical Studies: International Journal of Psychoanalysis, 2* (2), 1–22.

Winnicott, D (1986). *Home is where we start from, Essays by a psycho-analyst.* W.W. Norton.

Winnicott, DW (1971). *Playing and reality.* Routledge Press.

Winnicott, DW (1975). The manic defence. In *Through Pediatrics to Psycho-Analysis*, (pp. 262–277). New York: Basic Books. (Original work published 1935)

Wilcox, HC, Arria, AM, Caldeira, KM, Vincent, KB, Pinchevsky, GO, O'Grady, KE (2010). Prevalence and predictors of persistent suicide ideation, plans and attempts during college. *Journal of Affective Disorders, 127* (1–3), 287–294. 10.1016/j.jad.2010.04.017

Yeats, WB (1962). Vacillation. In ML Rosenthal (Ed.), *Selected poems and two plays of William Butler Yeats* (pp. 134–137). Collier Books. (Original work published 1932).

Chapter 6

Treating Trauma in the Fishbowl of University and College Counseling Centers[1]

Introduction

The ubiquity of trauma in everyday life ensures that most therapists, regardless of professional degree (i.e., Ph.D., Psy.D., LCSW, LMHC, etc.) have experience in treating it. This is certainly true for clinicians working in university and college counseling centers (UCCs), as trauma is highly prevalent in adolescents and young adults of college age (Saunders & Adams, 2014). Although, there is abundant writing about treating trauma, some of which we will discuss, we think it is noteworthy that we have been unable to find any published papers about doing so within institutions of higher education.[2] While it is safe to say that there are large areas of overlap with treating traumas in different contexts, in this chapter we discuss what is unique about its treatment within a university and college context.

An overview of what trauma is and some of its impacts

There are two primary mechanisms of trauma. The first is when we are exposed to a sudden unexpected incident that overwhelms our self-system and causes us to suffer intense physical and/or emotional pain. The second occurs when we are in a threatening situation for an extended period of time. According to the noted trauma psychiatrist, Bessel van der Kolk, "traumatization occurs when both internal and external resources are inadequate to cope with external threat" (1989, p. 393). In other words, individuals can become traumatized both by singular overwhelming events and by ongoing threats that they lack

DOI: 10.4324/9781003246558-7

resources to cope with. Speaking of trauma in general, the psycho-analyst James Grotstein poignantly says that what is traumatic to us is that which occurs to us before we have "imagined, phantasied, created, or 'autochtohonized' it" (2000, p. 45). We can be traumatized by what we cannot prepare for through imagination. And of course, when we are in the throes of trauma our ability to prepare is grossly impaired. Notably, trauma is subjective, not all people in equivalent situations will become traumatized.[3]

While both of these definitions highlight the external dimension that traumatic incidents and situations entail, Webb and Widseth (2009) describe situations whereby trauma seems to occur through more internal means. They distinguish between traumas with a sense of agency and those without. For the latter, we typically feel traumatized by external events, such as natural disasters or being assaulted. Whereas in the former, we feel (accurately or not) that we are responsible for what has happened. These include times when we feel we have acted in ways that conflict with how we otherwise see ourselves. These are actions which in his poem, *Vacillation*, William Butler Yeats (1932, unnumbered) says, appall our "conscience" or "vanity" in some fundamental way whether or not we have done harm to another person (but, of course, most typically reflecting those times when we have). Our understanding of this kind of trauma is complicated further if we consider agency within our appreciation of reenactment. Here, we act from the place of an internalized aggressor. We act in hurtful ways and even feel responsible for what has happened even if we do so only with sparse realization of the historical train of agency that is at play. About such trauma and the complex mix of agency and enactment, we will say more later.

Since trauma speaks to an experience of being overwhelmed by threats to our sense of self, being and ongoingness, there is nothing per se that is pathological about it. When traumatized we react to protect ourselves through a series of psychological and physiological mechanisms referred to as "fight, flight or freeze," any or all of which we engage to mitigate the effects of the traumatic event so that we can protect our very being and self-integrity.

However, when we are unable effectively to fight, flee or freeze and are thus overwhelmed, we are at real risk of becoming traumatized. Whether stemming from discrete instance(s) or ongoing cumulation, trauma can generate learned helplessness, difficulties modulating affect attention-focusing issues, and problems with remembering old information and the processing of new information (Bloom, 1999). Moreover, in the face of trauma, we may dissociate or disconnect from our current experiences leaving us susceptible to later traumatic reenactment. Not surprisingly, trauma negatively impacts not just our psyches but also our bodies, leaving us more vulnerable to all forms of illness and suffering.

While trauma impacts us directly it also ripples out into how we present ourselves in our immediate and local communities. As survivors of trauma, we have to deal with a world that feels decidedly unsafe and this greatly influences how we relate to self and other. In situations that traumatize us, we are neither able to anchor it within the structure of already available symbolic encoding (our pre-conceptions or "imagination"; Grotstein, 2000) nor able to create adequate, new foundation for encoding it within words (new conceptions). We are, in a sense, stuck in "no man's land." This leaves us highly susceptible to utilizing indirect means to communicate and, at times, to enact unconsciously what we have experienced. This can be disruptive to local contexts, especially when those contexts are unprepared to receive these communications from trauma-informed locations. When this happens, confusion, anger and a host of other feelings ensue in a predominating way.

These ripples are often magnified in university and college communities. These communities are an interesting blend of being both an "open" and "closed" context. Working within it often feels like being in or around a "fishbowl." The privacy of the closed context is always being negotiated through the variably transparent or translucent glass that distinguishes whether we are situated *in* the bowl as the *observed* or *outside* of it as the *observer*. As a result of this, communication of information is refracted in ways that can feel unpredictable, unreliable and unmodulated. This is especially important to keep in mind when we are treating traumatized students. When we do so, we are *in* the fishbowl with the student but *are* so without the student's freedom to leave the bowl when we wish.

Some aspects of the university and college as "fishbowl"

An example of the fishbowl effect occurs when students, inspired by the communitarian ideals about sharing and the importance of social relationships, share deeply personal matters with various community members. This can include roommates and classmates, coaches, professors and advisors. Sometimes, what are shared are their treatment experiences at the counseling center. Then and especially when there is overt suffering, these good-hearted people may offer advice or try to help out in a way that creates a situation of "too many cooks in the kitchen." While well-intentioned, this truly can complicate the treatment; the relational field (Stern, 2009, 2015, 2018) expands to include all sorts of what in the relatively "closed context" of a traditional therapy would be considered extra-therapeutic contacts. Thus, in the fishbowl context of the university or college counseling center what is *extra* to the treatment becomes often enough that which is *typical* to it.

Sometimes in the close-at-hand and omnipresent social network that exists on many campuses, experiences pertinent to the trauma can be readily exacerbated or recapitulated. Not only can this be upsetting for others with their own traumatic history but also it can activate protective responses on the part of the university or college. And these pressures parlay into pressure on the therapist to offer treatment which prioritizes amelioration of symptoms over resolution of the conflicts of being-ness which create them.

For example, institutions generate and maintain all forms of support systems, such as Behavioral Intervention Teams (BIT) designed with good intentions to monitor students and keep key figures in the loop. These efforts can be sometimes very helpful but at other times an unwitting interference in the treatment. This happens when the "team" for whatever reason becomes acutely aware of its own fishbowl situated-ness and of having to be the embodiment of the institution's accepted role (usually of being a bountiful and nurturant caregiver). In response to the pressure that accompanies *being observed* in this role, the "team" makes clear the it is *observing* the therapist-fish. Within the fishbowl, then, the therapist can feel eyes that plead "doing something urgently" to make things better for the student. In the most problematic iterations of this dynamic, patience with working through conflicts central to the trauma is compromised, and our understanding that trauma reflects the effects of unmodulated action gets lost in thinking that unmodulated action will "fix" it.

Notably, while BIT teams and other such interventions are often designed to prevent this type of situation, it is the nature of trauma for it to be created despite our best efforts. This means that we as therapists always have to listen for extra-observers and try to reckon, if possible, *with* the student how being observed can impact the treatment process itself. Of course, this is not always easy or even possible. After all, that trauma grows out of an event denied "imagination" (anticipation) logically portends treatment difficulties in creating and maintaining space for imagination.

Multiple self-state models and our understanding of trauma

Before discussing the effects of the fishbowl nature of higher education on the treatment of trauma within UCCs, we must first say a little bit about how we think about the self and subjectivity and what happens during traumatic experiences. We especially want to highlight the processes of dissociation and enactment, which are central to understanding and treating trauma.

A confluence of theories

We think the views that we describe below sit comfortably alongside and compliment the positions of existential-relational situated-ness we have described throughout this book. Up to this point, we have focused more exclusively on developmental processes that we associate with the positions which differentially delineate how we are situated with respect to otherness and our experience of agency. While we have discussed instances where we may become "stuck" in one of these positions and noted that this may result from traumatic experience, we have cast a broad net to underline that movement between the existential-relational positions is a part of everyday living where such stuck-ness is more temporary than otherwise. However, here where we specifically consider trauma, we need to take a more in-depth look at how more contemporary views of self, informed by trauma theory, describe the processes of emergent identity and what happens when there is trauma.

Similar to our perspective, these contemporary views challenge the ideas of an isolated, integrated Cartesian self. They emphasize, instead, that from infancy onward our burgeoning sense of self is fragmented, i.e., incongruous, multiple and so at times in-cohesive and not necessarily linked to other self-experiences. These nuanced theories of how subjectivity emerges from these multiple relationships shed light on the normative ways we protect ourselves (i.e., dissociation) and come to know variously unknown self-states (i.e., enactment). An appreciation of these protective adaptations is crucial to our understanding of how to treat trauma within the uniqueness of campus communities.

The multiplicity of self

> In reality ... every ego, so far from being a unity is in the highest degree a manifold world, a constelled heaven, a chaos of forms, of states and stages, of inheritances and potentialities. It appears to be a necessity as imperative as eating and breathing for everyone to be forced to regard this chaos as a unity and to speak of his ego as though it were a one-fold and clearly detached and fixed phenomenon. Even the best of us shares the delusion. (1929, p. 79)

The above quote from Herman Hesse's novel, *Steppenwolf*, which was first published in English in 1929, anticipates by many years contemporary perspectives of the self, informed by psychoanalysis (Sullivan, 1950, 1956; Stern, 2004, 2006; Bromberg, 1993, 1994, 1998, 2003), trauma theory (Chefetz & Bromberg, 2004; Bailey & Brand, 2017; Kluft, 1985, 1991) and dialogical self-theory (Janet, 1888; Hermans & Kempen, 1993; Hermans, 2001). These perspectives consider dissociation and enactment as expectable ways of dealing with our emerging sense and experience of ourselves as fundamentally embodied and constituted by our relational and cultural situation(s) (Bromberg, 1994). Following these perspectives, we might think of our "self" as a network of various self-states, each of which is coherent within specific contexts and situations. In this, each self-state may be thought of as a developing "being" and so situated along the continuum we have offered. As described by Philip Bromberg (1993), "Self-experience originates in relatively unlinked self-states, *each coherent in its own right*, and the experience of being a unitary self is an acquired, developmentally adaptive illusion" (p. 162, our emphasis).

This coherence we can understand to be as simple as the different ways we act when we are with mother or father; at school in a classroom or playing at recess and so forth. The multiplicity of self-states, in other words, is something we understand to reflect the variety of relationships among our social states of being-ness. And these varieties of social me's are comprised both of our awareness of how significant other's see us and of our more agentic private "I" (Mead, 1967; Marková, 2003a, 2003b; James, 1890/1950; Sullivan, 1950, 1953; Hermans, 2001) that is developing concurrently.

The social "me"

Our sense of the social "me" develops through our social interactions with important others. If we locate this within our framework of existential-relational positions, we might say these others begin as "non-me's" (or "not-me's" when we are in the paranoid-schizoid position). With the passage of time and more social interactions we achieve more semiotic capacities and these non-me's (or not-me's) become "you's." Relationship with "you" in turn informs how "you" see "me." Hence, my sense of "me" encapsulates "my" internalization of other people's attitudes toward and about "me."

Existing both within our own minds as well as that of others speaks to our experiences of our burgeoning sense of self as fractured. The "me" in relationship to mother while eating is different than the "me" in relationship to her while playing; to say nothing of the "me" that interacts with father. "Me" develops through the reflected appraisals and ruptures with our significant others' – both conscious and un-conscious – such that the burgeoning infant rather quickly under-stands "good-me" to be pleasing to others and "bad-me" to be displeasing and a source of anxiety (Sullivan, 1953). Notably, then "me" encapsulates "you" both in a very specific way; but also, ac-cording to George Herbert Mead (1967) a very social way. Through taking actions and playing roles – say police and robbers – children develop a variety of senses of selves.

Although complicating things a bit further, it is important to note that our sense of "me" is limited in that we can never know truly and fully how Others see us. That we exist in the mind of an "Other" is, on the one hand, liberating – we can be free from the confines of our own minds, but it also can be terrifying. We lack true control over our sense of "being"; we are always, in a sense, in state of discombobulating alienation from our illusion of being an essential "self" (Sullivan, 1950).

The private "I"

Our sense of "me" begins to inform our experience of ourselves as an agentic and private "I." Drawing from Vygotsky (1978), we agree that the basis of our experiences are social. In his words, "every function in the child's cultural development appears twice: First, on the social level and later, on the individual level; first, between people (interpsycholoigcal) and then inside the child (intrapsychological" (p. 57). This constitutes our immediate familial culture and our ever-broadening societal structures. Notably, in a way similar to our grasp on our "me," our sense of ourselves as "I" is also limited. We can only grasp imperfectly an ongoing self through the relationship between our "I" and "me."

What we are able to grasp in this interaction develops into a more private experience of ourselves as active and agentic. Our experience of becoming an "I" develops through others' reactions, especially through the symbolic activities entailed in our "naming" and "un-naming" of our initial actions. As noted throughout this book, this is crucial. Our ability to be reflective agents emerges as a result of our activity in the world, which has to be interpreted by others in meaningful ways (Zittoun & Gillespie, 2015; Gillespie, 2005).

Given the sometimes clumsy and aggressive swoop of our *becoming*, we can misattribute in our conceptions of development (as we have discussed in Chapter 4) when our agency comes into play. We must hold in mind that we are reliant upon key Others to help us develop our capacity to be a reflective and agentic "I." They do this through their tolerance then embrace of our desire to "name" ourselves (and others). In other words, we need the sanction of our caregivers to be multiple "me's" in different situations and contexts so that we can begin to name and un-name ourselves. When we are restricted from this and the "me" that can be only that which "you" allow, our burgeoning agency can be delimited in truly consequential ways. In these cases, aspects of our experience that important Others cannot tolerate or symbolize may develop as "not-me" parts of ourselves. They are inaccessible to "I" through conscious thought. Thus, "I" and "me" are dynamically entwined, whereby "me" reflects more outward-facing social relationships and "I" stands in reaction to them, more personal and private – but still social through relationship to "me."

As we have noted, when things go well and our relational field is reasonably rich, safe and stable, we become able to engage in the world in meaningful and fulfilling ways. "I" and "me" interact with each other creatively; we can move fluidly between different self-states and play with similarity and difference. However, when things are problematic or where the significant Others in our life cannot meet our needs "good enough," we struggle. Trauma instantiates particular challenges to development especially in our early years – though these challenges can occur at any point in life if we are traumatized. Accordingly, we want to describe some of the other unique ways we may be traumatized, begin to protect ourselves from trauma, and then enact traumas as a way of beginning to work them through.

Challenges of development

Dissociation

In thinking about the trauma of early childhood, we begin with the defensive processes of dissociation. In earlier days of clinical theory, dissociation was considered something we automatically employed to regulate our emotional responses, when extreme events overwhelmed the internal and external resources available to us for coping. In other words, the prevailing view was that when threatening situations severely compromise our emotional and physiological capacities to sooth and self-regulate, our body and mind automatically protected itself by disconnecting from conscious connection with the ongoing (or anticipated) experience.

Over time, dissociation went from being something considered extreme and pathological to being understood as an unconscious defense which exists on a continuum. We all dissociate to some extent. How much we distance ourselves from our immediate situation varies from "checking out" to briefly distancing ourselves, perhaps by feeling outside our bodies, floating above ourselves and looking down. Of course, where on the continuum we fall on the continuum is contingent upon how threatened we feel.

In its normative sense, dissociation helps us to manage the potential overwhelming angst that comes from vulnerability and anxiety as we move through different aspects of our daily lives. For instance, as we move between familial relationships or between school and home, we may dissociate versions of ourselves with the result that our school self is very different than our at home self. In this regard, we foreground one aspect of self and background other aspects of ourselves. This is clearly adaptive as it allows us to focus upon the context at hand and not bring into situations ways of being that may conflict. Furthermore, this creates a cohesive feeling of self.

This normal experience of dissociation is contrasted with times when dissociation is more urgently required as protection against traumatic experience. These are experiences that threaten affectively and/or physiologically to overwhelm our sense of security and stability. These can be acutely traumatic situations that are manifestly visible, such as a robbery, rape or assault. Traumatic situations, however, can also be relatively opaque. We can find ourselves in a situation which can be "triggering." This is a situation which, although perhaps not noticeable to an outside observer, threatens the overall safety and security of our self-system (the illusion of a singular self) because it stirs up aspects of ourselves that we have deemed unsafe and cordoned off (i.e., the not-me selves). For instance, when we are faced with experiences that harken back to the abandonment we felt because of the failure of an early caregiver to symbolize our experience, we may dissociate as a defense against experiencing the overwhelming feelings of fear and pain. Dissociating in its various forms (derealization, depersonalization, denial, avoidance, etc.) are all ways essentially of retreating from what is unbearable to keep as much of the self as possible feeling protected and secure (Chefetz & Bromberg, 2004).

Returning to the words of Bromberg (1993), when faced with trauma,

[T]his illusion of unity is ... threatened with unavoidable, precipitous disruption that it becomes in itself a liability, because it is in jeopardy of being overwhelmed by input it cannot process symbolically and deal with as a state of conflict.

As a defense, then, dissociation leads to almost a literal stop in making associations to (or meanings for) our experience; a sort of zoning out, ignoring or not paying attention, especially to experiences that are flooding us with intense anxiety and fear.

Clinically, when therapist (or patient) observes something, say "You seem jealous of so and so" to which, the other says "I had not considered that," we find evidence of dissociation. We can conclude that experience of jealousy is somehow threatening the continuous sense of self and, therefore, is dissociated. Of course, there can be many reasons why the experience is threatening – perhaps the patient's father became jealous of the attention the patient received from mother as an infant/child and the patient's conscious embrace of this awareness was too threatening. Similarly, when patients express affect, such as crying (but really any affect) without being aware that they are crying (not to mention why), we begin to wonder what experience is being dissociated. More extreme are times when talking about something ordinary triggers a strong explosive response or when talking about something painful causes the patient to almost flatten out as if they are no longer present.

In this respect, dissociation is embedded within the structure of our psyche (Bromberg, 1993). It is not enough to have dissociated within a situation; the self has to remain alert for future threatening instances. The self employs dissociation structurally almost as an early alarm system that is constantly vigilant and on-guard. This protects the self, but it does so at high cost. Dissociated aspects of the self-remain unsymbolized (or unformulated in the language of Donnel Stern, 2004, 2009, 2018) and can even remain unavailable to symbolization. If so, they are unintegrated and split off and then unconsciously are encoded as "not-me" states.

Take, for example, this patient's dream about her family soon after the, death of her father. In the dream, her brother (Jim) gets hit by a bus that comes out of nowhere. The patient has to tell her parents (J.D. and Meg) about the accident, but it turns out that the parents already know it happened, although do not know the details. Ten or fifteen minutes into associations to the dream, the patient looks up and says to the therapist that her father's name was James. She then remarks that the names in the dream, Jim and J.D., are both nick-names of her father. Her knowledge of this had been dissociated at the time until it hit like a bus. We then talked about the care-taking role she took on immediately in the face of the loss and whether that action allowed space for mourning.

Within our campus communities we might recognize dissociation when a reading in class triggers a strong and surprising emotional reaction in a student. We might also "see" dissociation when someone suddenly starts behaving or acting differently in class or in meetings. For instance, a successful student starts doing poorly or someone who is usually well kempt appears more disheveled. In these cases, when we share what we have noticed, the person, even if they recognize that something has significantly changed, is at a loss to explain why it has changed.

Dissociation is a blunt instrument. In an effort to protect a sense of integrity and self, large swaths of self-experience may not be observed or interacted with. There is thus a sense of a lack of awareness of what caused the upset or an emotional reaction. Frequently, these patients express a vague feeling of something being wrong but cannot string together a cogent narrative of the source of the pain. On the flip side, there can be hyper-vigilance. A type of constant awareness which cannot be turned off. This can leave one feeling continuously overwhelmed and triggered as if there is no escape. Also, the need to pay exquisite at-tention to a situation ensures that the forest is missed for the trees.

The insidiousness is clear. The self does not respond to threats by locating them outside the self; rather, internally the threat is asso-ciated with certain self-states, certain ways of being, that are too emotionally overwhelming and therefore cut off. They, in other words, are subject to amnesia; existing and being forgotten rather than being repressed (Bromberg, 1993; Stein, 2001).

Enactments and vicious cycles

Being cut off from our experience means we lose access to our emotional states as well as possibly to the memories and cognitions that correspond to those states. This in turn impacts our abilities to make decisions, to exercise foresight and to navigate effectively the world. This can lead to a type of dissociative enactment whereby individuals unknowingly place themselves in harmful but familiar situations. This is understood as both the pull of the familiar that gives off a false sense of safety and also the unconscious hope to have a different and therefore less traumatic experience. This apparent paradox of acting in ways that may further our experience of trauma is a hallmark of traumatic reenactment; it reflects a way of expressing dissociated thoughts and feelings (Rosenbaum & Webb, 2019).

Enactment comes about from the multiplicity of our self-system. Thus, while the self learns to dissociate for protection, we remain social and comprised of "I" and "me" states. Recall how our sense of "I" developed out of thinking about one's reactions to other's responses. This does not stop just because areas of the self are cordoned off as "not-me." Rather, these parts of ourselves, continue to seek recognition except they do so through alternative means, "enactments," which are usually but not always best characterized as action rather than word-based in their expression (Stern, 2004; Aron, 2003; Bass, 2003).

Not surprisingly, these enactments are a result of having much of one's inner world dominated by a defensive structure meant to avoid potentially harmful situations and prevent painful experiences. Hence, they are verbal and non-verbal behavioral patterns that occur outside of conscious awareness and intent (Stern, 2004; Levenson, 1983/2005). Of course, everyone enacts aspects of experience that they are not aware of. Think here, for instance, about being told that you've behaved in a certain way that you did not realize and that you then acknowledge is true. Similarly, think of the common experience of a patient saying something then commenting that they had no intention of saying what they said. In any case, the pernicious effect of trauma is that it promotes enactments which often entail engagement in expression that is unsafe and potentially retraumatizing. Without the mediation of new meaning-making through the use of language, the paradox of seeking to *repeat in order to redo* (fix) almost always ends *in repeat which only repeats* (hurts again).

This makes sense if we stop to think about it. When we are traumatized, we live with significant gaps ("not-me") in the range of our experiences that we can symbolize and use for making meaning. Dissociation limits our perceptual field and ability to recognize important aspects of situations, both internally (feelings, mood states, motivations, etc.) and externally in such a way that we are unmediated; we are relegated consequentially to being either *hypersensitive* or *insensitive* in our discernment of the danger of situations. Indeed, what is often being enacted is precisely this lack of knowledge about our inner and external worlds for keeping ourselves safe. As a result, individuals who are traumatized are at greater risk for new trauma than others (Kessler et al., 2010), especially when the "insensitive" aspect prevails.

It is a perfect storm of vicious cycles. Trauma leads to the felt need to be safe, generating conditions that are, in fact, often more dangerous and the cause of more trauma. In this respect, enactments also become one way in which others, not just therapists, learn about the presence of trauma and dissociated self-states. Take this common experience. A patient and therapist have a difficult session, one where the therapist feels uncomfortable afterward for reasons, they cannot quite name. At the next session, the patient talks about going out afterward and engaging in impulsive risky behavior. The therapist understands this as a reaction to something in the session that could not be symbolically discussed and so had to be enacted.

As therapists, then, we try to juggle a variety of sensibilities. We try to keep ourselves aware of indices of dissociation so that we can link these to various self-states but also thinking about ongoing relational processes. Relatedly, we also have to maintain a conviction that dissociative enactments are brought about by both historic and contemporary "triggers." For patients who dissociate there is often difficulty recalling what happened within their immediate context, the semiotic ground as it were, to have initiated dissociation. Enactment signals that something has happened, but working with patients to convey the belief that it is about something within their more immediate field can take time and effort. We approach these discussions with a keen attention to our sense of our connection to the patient so that we can tune ourselves to what can be invited into symbolic expression and what still feels off limits (too threatening). "The 'content' that is traumatic is embedded in our relational experience of patient (that is itself part of the content), and this unsymbolized relational experience is re-lived by being enacted repeatedly between us and the patient as an intrinsic part of their relationship" (Chefetz & Bromberg, 2004) until time and careful work allows for its fuller mediation in the world of words.

In short, in order to become known, processed, and worked through, the unsymbolized self-states must be enacted within a therapeutic relationship where not only these states can be cognitively known, but more important (and so more difficultly) affectively re-experienced, so they can be symbolized in different (safer) ways. It is not enough for us and our patient and to *talk through* what happened; in a real way, the patient must experience our care and concern and also feel and tolerate the emotions that had been dissociated. Within the therapeutic relationship the way we come to know the patient hinges, then, on not just be told information but on experiencing *along with* the patient.

A colleague (name removed) shared the following vignette about working with a patient she called Elizabeth, who initially presented to the center as a freshman with difficulties maintaining her relationship with her boyfriend of five years. She appeared confident and self-sufficient, coming from an affluent and well-off family. Her apparent dependence on the boyfriend confused the therapist until sometime during the second year of treatment. Then, the patient when talking about her relationship issues revealed significant family problems. Her father had a long history of health issues, which absorbed most of his time and financial resources in the search for successful treatment. More recently, mom who had been "downsized" lost her job and had turned toward alcohol to help cope. These issues had been displaced (and so dissociated) into the current boyfriend relationship, which it turned out was the most stable relationship in the patient's life.

As the therapy progressed into the patient's junior year, the therapist and patient worked to witness and tolerate the gradual family disintegration. The parents divorced, each medical procedure for father felt like life or death, and mom's alcoholism went untreated. Patient and therapist felt helpless as every intervention failed. Suddenly, at one-point listening to the patient talk about mom's sulking, the therapist burst out, "Grow Up!" While intended for mother, the enactment of the normally quieter and more reserved therapist signaled an important moment in treatment which allowed both her and the patient to talk more fully about the mother's dependence upon the patient, her needs to be in that position, and what separating would look like. Moreover, the patient experienced her therapist's real care in response to her despondency.

Thus, dissociation and enactment – the attempt of the patient (and analyst) to bring to consciousness parts of the self that have been dissociated – are central to understanding trauma and its sequela. From our perspective, while both dissociation and enactment occur for many of the patients we see in our offices, they are most important in helping us understand trauma, traumatic reactions and its treatment within college contexts.

Some considerations about agency

The complicated nature of trauma, dissociation and enactment has consequences for how we think about traumas and for the extent to which we think trauma involves a sense of agency (Webb & Widseth, 2009). Broadly speaking, this differentiation is used to distinguish between traumas that in effect happen to us, such as a natural disaster or even a physical assault, and those where we feel a sense of complicity, i.e., a soldier who has killed someone. Dissociation, however, blurs this distinction.

Frequently, in these cases, patients talk about the sense of being complicit in the creation of circumstances, which generates and causes ongoing trauma. They describe a vague awareness of being pulled by some version of themselves toward doing something that can potentially be harmful or damaging to the rest of themselves. However, they also in a real way cannot seem to stop themselves. Through the beauty of literary expression John Steinbeck, without explicit acknowledgment of the unconscious, "knows" this, saying in *East of Eden:* "Sometimes a man wants to be stupid if it lets him do a thing his cleverness forbids" (1992, p. 254).

This leaves them in the worst of double binds. Feeling victimized – but by themselves. In these moments of extreme shame and humiliation, they thus feel as if they've transgressed morally – similar to those who experience trauma with a sense of agency but also feel helpless to have stopped it. When seen from the vantage point of enactment however, these traumas outline precisely the relational dynamic often at play. As young children, these patients have known what might generate a terrible response in the caretaking other; however, their needs to also be loved and cared for would have drawn them into enacting certain forms of conduct with the hope of having some of their needs met but more often than not the experience of being abandoned, left or even hurt.

A woman student presented to the counseling center with a history of sexual abuse by a brother. This was a brother who was jealous of her being the apple of their mother's eye while both of them, him and her, suffered from a taciturn, work-obsessed and physically absent father. Complicating her history further was that she was raped in high school by a family friend. In her therapy, she spoke of how liberated she felt to leave a home where she had felt so deeply un-protected by those who were supposed to be safe and loving. She had resolved in college to have a "new start" and to "fix this" by finding a romantic partner who would be protective of her. An upper-class student who was in "law enforcement" studies seemed like the ticket to her. However, one year into that relationship she realized that this man's apparent self-assurance and certainty about right and wrong was the cover for deep uncertainties about being worthy and for bitter resentments about how he had felt unfairly treated by loved ones. His anxieties manifested in an intransigent need to control her behavior and nearly paranoid fears of being cheated on. After several episodes of her partner "losing it," having raging outbursts where he belittled her because she couldn't do anything right, she realized with deep regret that she had "gone from the pot to the frying pan." Looking back on her relationship to this man she felt guilty for having been so "stupid" in pursuing a romance with him. In the early stages of getting to know him the man had told her how angry and hurt he was by the rejection of a previous romance, and in the context of telling her this story he had sought to elicit from her a promise that she would "never ever do that" to him. Reflecting in her therapy about this, the woman said she "sort of knew" that she should have walked away from the relationship before it deepened further. However, there was a special appeal to her in this man's combination of deep vulnerability, that she didn't want to extinguish, and his "strength" of opinion, that she took for safety, that compelled her decision to give the romance a try.

We might then begin to think of agency with something like brackets around it, representable as [agency]. Patients, who have been traumatized and begin to develop awareness of their various self-states, struggle to hold the various parts of themselves in something like a comprehensive fashion. It would be mistaken to say or think as if they lack any choice or agency but similarly mistaken to consider them a free agent. Instead, they exist somewhere along a continuum where some days and in some situations, more may be accessible and other days and situations less. Not only does this make their lives feel highly unpredictable and chaotic – these patients describe literally not only knowing what tomorrow will bring or even the next hour or two (Stein, 2001). But this too gets enacted so that the people around them, whether friends, therapists or family may feel equally confused and chaotic.

It should begin to be clear that these types of patients pose a unique challenge to colleges and universities where they are often living in situations that on the one hand may be some of the most secure and stable in their lives and on the other hand are also incredibly fluid, unstable and changing. In this regard, note the seductive and therein highly problematic message that institutes of higher education often convey to students: "Come and bring all of yourself to us. This is a safe space for growth. However, do not get too comfortable, because you are only here for a few years (whereas the institution is here forever and its faculty/administrator for longer). Moreover, as we alluded to earlier, its fishbowl nature ensures that bumps rather than be smoothed over may also be magnified and exacerbated. With this in mind, let us now turn to talk about the treatment of trauma on university and college campuses.

The complexities of providing treatment in the fishbowl

As we alluded to at the start of this chapter, the dual facets of trauma, dissociation and enactment create unique challenges for treating students, especially those with trauma in our environments of higher education. The unconscious pull of traumatic reenactment and the painful nature of the affects experienced make it difficult to "sit" with difficult feelings, a necessary requisite of therapy. "Sitting with" allows for the mentation, or the development of symbolic meaning and eventual integration within the acceptable range of one's sense of self of these feelings. Alternatively, acting out serves to sustain the early trauma.

However, what happens frequently enough, especially early on in treatment when feelings may be stirred up, is that feelings are expressed in ambiguous silence or a displaced way that the therapist does not decipher. When this happens, which is often an enactment in and of itself (around the patient's needs not being met and their inability to express them), the potential for other or further enactment is high. These enactments can draw the attention of others and lead to all sorts of extra-therapeutic contacts that then have to be contended with in the treatment or can threaten the treatments' integrity.

The influence of others

Living in close proximity to peers who may have had good experiences with other therapists or know of friends who have had bad experiences with a particular therapist can lead to suggestions to change to a different therapist when immediate relief is not found. Similarly, faculty, coaches, and administrators in their desire to be helpful may suggest alternative therapies or approaches. While these efforts are almost always supportive and designed to alleviate suffering, they often involve an action, namely leaving the "world of words."

This chance increases in an environment or community where such inability of the therapist to give immediate relief can be viewed as some kind of incompetence: inadequate training about a specific problem or insensitivity to the particularities of some culture or racial group. We hasten to say that this explanation of incompetence or insensitivity is not something that we think should be foreclosed from consideration.

At times, these suggestions gain urgency when a student continues to do poorly, whether within academics, social or athletic spheres (to name a few). In these cases, issues arising from students having confided in others become sources of system-wide worry, anxiety and frustration. The need to "fix" or "resolve" a complex trauma so some desired outcome can get on track generates pressure within the system, oftentimes with minimal outlet. Indeed, sometimes the therapy room is the only "safe place" removed from such pressures, which in the face of outside influence can begin to enact the feeling of pressure. Thus, a concerned coach reaching out to the therapist to "check in" and see "how they can help," while certainly well intentioned communicates quite a bit about the situation.

Clinical example

One student-client with a history of fractured connection with his father allowed himself to connect deeply with his male therapist during his senior year. As graduation and the likely end of the therapy relationship approached, however, this brilliant student's attendance in class and his performance in class began to slip. A dean, who had been following the student carefully over the years and who knew via the student's candor that the student was in therapy at the counseling center, called up the service's director to share her concern about the student. She added that she had recently seen the student wandering unkempt and "smelly" around campus with his sleeping bag draped around his shoulders. In this situation, because the director and this dean had a weather-tested relationship of mutual respect and trust, the director was able, without sharing specific knowledge of the therapy's status and his conversations about this with the therapist, to reassure the dean that the public behavior being witnessed, while alarming, was something that had to run its course and that it was something which was expectable given that the student was investing himself as highly in the therapy as he did typically with his academics.

In short, the director was able to say that the dean was witnessing an enactment of issues and a dissociation of feelings that were emerging in the therapy relationship. This reassured the dean of his confidence that with patience, although not without consequences, the acting out would find its containment again in the therapy relationship; and that the student-client was not in an uncontrolled pre-psychotic spiral downward.

Community anxieties: Institute "not-me" self-states

This situation speaks to additional challenges in the treatment of students who have been traumatized, specifically, the need of the therapist and counseling center to hold not only the students' anxieties but also the institutes at large (Slochower, 2004). While almost always arising from sympathetic ears and good-intentioned conscious feelings, institutional efforts at "repair" are also enactments. Indeed, often underlying these efforts are "not-me" feelings of the "helper," such as helplessness, despair, anger or terror.

More broadly, students with histories of trauma may trigger Institutional "not-me's" as well. In these cases, as enactments unfold the institution may find itself in the role of "bad one." While being in this role is sufficiently jarring to the institution that there is pressure to view the student's reaction as transference or projection, it is important, at least for the clinician to acknowledge and grapple with the very real harm an institution may, intentional or not, perpetuate. For example, "harmless oversights," such as not having appropriate structures in place for helping, for example, international and first-generation students feel comfortable and safe can also be seen as "not-me" enactments on the part of the institution in their non-malicious failure to consider what all their students need.

Indeed, the strength of the pressure/demand for relief is so strong that it is not just members of the community outside of the consulting room who are sometimes quick to suggest that arising frustration be soothed with some determined "action." A significant number of counseling centers (including the one where the first author practices) have adopted policies of "no questions asked" if a student-client wants to make a change of therapist. In other words, counseling centers and clinicians have their own "not-me" states, which can be brought into enactment. While this might be an understandable and adaptive policy for a center to adopt if it wants to be viewed with positive regard in communities, which so adamantly herald their ethos of acceptance and validation of others, it is, nonetheless, a policy which elides funda-mental good sense about the process of working through the com-plexities inherent to dissociation and enactment. Or, in this case sitting (or at the very least encouraging a session) with the potential bad and not-me feelings that arise from trying to put into words the thoughts and feelings about what is not working with a particular therapist.

Helping colleges and counseling centers navigate trauma

Keeping this in mind, we now turn to some thoughts about how UCCs can help their institution navigate the ways traumatic enactments, particularly when they draw from the "not-me" self-states of key figures and the institution as a whole. Take the following (not so uncommon) student-client situation:

Frank, a male junior, who was at a critical junction in the therapy work got drunk over the weekend and in a fight with his girlfriend angrily broke with his fist a glass window in her dorm. A vigorous debate then ensued in the presence of the dean between the counseling center therapist (who was granted freedom to break confidentiality by his student-client) and the supervisor of the security officer who had been the first responder in the incident. The security supervisor viewed the action by the student as violence which warranted removal from residence either by hospitalization or by being sent home. The supervisor volunteered that she had a sister who was a rape survivor and that she herself had been prompted by this and her role on campus to get certified as a rape counselor.

The therapist, after talking to the student profitably enough to puzzle about what was being enacted by his behavior, both in terms of a repetition of childhood trauma and in terms of a plea in the relationship with the therapist to intervene, so to demonstrate her caring, expressed her opinion that hospitalization would offer the student no useful treatment and that the action was not likely to be repeated and so sending the student home not necessary. In fact, the therapist was able to argue that sending the student away, either to a hospital or to "home," would repeat a kind of abandonment by caretakers that was central to the student's trauma.

The dean, of course, was put in a very difficult position. How could he accept one of the opinions of his staff without making the other feel disrespected? This was a dilemma, which in and of itself had parallels in the early trauma of the student who was often placed in "choice" situations, situations where his parents had to choose between different versions of a story as offered by him and his older sister. The student was often disbelieved by his parents in deference to that sister. The dean in this situation, again a savvy one, allowed the conversation among him, the therapist, and the security supervisor to play out without a pressure for a snap decision. Ultimately, the supervisor agreed to the student staying in residence if the therapist would sign off, take full responsibility for the decision, and if the college would put on record her, the supervisor's disagreement with that decision.

The role of the counseling center in holding "not-me" anxieties

This example is emblematic of the chaos and anxiety that can be generated in these situations of trauma enactment. It also shows the important role the college therapist must play in understanding the dynamic process that is at hand with a client and the institution. In this regard, the therapist may find themselves as the middle person, having to communicate sensitively that process to the "fishbowl" so that the chaos and anxiety that is generated can be contained and also having to convey some of what is happening to their patient to help them navigate the immediate context. Given this, it often makes sense to split roles in ways that preserve and protect the counseling relationship. Accordingly, directors may wind up providing more communication with deans or student evaluations so that counselors can focus on treating their patients.

Notably, the systemic anxiety rises and tests the integration of the "not-me's" of key community players and the institution itself. If these players' anxiety is sufficiently high, the institutional response to the student's enactment can easily become an enactment, often one whose unconscious intent is to expel from reckoning any sense that we, the community, are anything but loving and caring. Preventing this reckoning often leads to an institutional response, which is imbalanced in either a phobic or counter-phobic way as regards toleration of excess. Hence, the excess demonstrated by the student's action leads to expulsion of the key player's "not-me's" by either insufficiently considered acceptance of the student's action or premature intolerance of it.

Given the chaotic and disruptive nature of trauma it is not surprising that there are also plenty of times when the counseling center cannot hold or contain its effects. When this happens, the counseling center may be "behind the train" frantically throwing down train tracks to prevent destruction or crash. For instance, if the counselor had been unable to discern the meaning of her student's enactment in the example described above, the situation may have gone very differently.

Similarly, there are also times where the counseling center is "destroyed" or allows for its destruction. Destruction ranges from almost the literal destroying of an essential function, such as being able to provide weekly psychotherapy (if that is how the mission is defined) or provide truly confidential treatment (Polychronis, 2018) to the more metaphorical. In the latter, when trauma stirs up campus-wide "not-me" self-states, which the center cannot hold, it may suffer a severe loss of face, and have to deal with a emergent "reputation" that "you cannot get helped there" or "that they don't care."

Here, trauma may be at both individual and macro levels, such that it would not be inappropriate to talk about a traumatic culture or toxic environment. The ability of the center to tolerate these attacks, whether true, unfounded, or more than likely a mixture of the two, and preserve its essential functions while tolerating and listening deeply to these attacks, provides a chance at meaning-making. Notably, survival does not mean capitulation to demands, either from students, deans, administrators, or otherwise that the center change or adapt different policies. While changes may happen, the center holds its role as collaborator in its willingness to change on some things but perhaps not with others. In this way, the center preserves its integrity and so its status as a possible partner for future students who've suffered trauma and require an intact enough interlocutor.

In this regard, the center being able to withstand attack and the inevitable feelings of disappointment and let-down, which arise from the realities of clinical work, helps to preserve the counseling space. This task often falls to Directors, Outreach Coordinators, and others who wear two hats. When trauma is at play, the chance for confusion and chaos is high and the pressure for quick fixes can make thinking difficult. We counsel here patience and tolerance and the belief that cooler heads usually prevail. This is crucial work. The outward "front of the house" needs to preserve and create safe therapy spaces "in the back of house." Indeed, the system sometimes may struggle so much to hold steady that it may be necessary for outside consultation and/or supervision to help maintain the integrity of center and clinician alike.

Summary

Trauma needs to be conceptualized and understood not as an individual's trauma (i.e., your's but not mine), but rather shared as ours. This does not mean that we lose sight that someone may be traumatized more acutely or recently than others. However, we may helpfully dissociate in such a way that we maintain our integrity to help a survivor of trauma (acute, chronic, ongoing, etc.) begin to cope and make meaning of their experience. Through considering trauma as shared, we allow space for the various self-states (patients, therapists, administrators, etc.) that we know will emerge during this work. This in turn, we think, provides the best chance at treating trauma within the unique eco-systems of Institutes of Higher Education.

Notes

1 A version of this chapter was published as Rosenbaum, P.J. & Webb, R.E. (2019). Treating trauma in the fishbowl of university and college counseling centers. *Journal of College Student Psychotherapy.* Online publication. https://doi.org/10.1080/87568225.2019.1671293

2 There are, of course, plenty of articles about Behavioral Intervention Teams, assessing trauma, preventing trauma, working with those who've been raped or sexually assaulted. However, to our knowledge, there is not a paper that talks broadly about what is unique about treating trauma within these institutions.

3 There is a lot to the specifics about trauma as it pertains to race, gender, sexuality, class and numerous other identifiers. While crucial to having a comprehensive understanding of trauma for the purpose of this memo, I focus broadly upon the devastating impact that trauma can have upon all of us.

References

Aron, L (2003). The paradoxical place of enactment in psychoanalysis: An introduction. *Psychoanalytic Dialogues, 13* (5), 623–631 10.1080/10481881309348760

Bailey, TD, & Brand, BL (2017). Traumatic dissociation: Theory, research and treatment. *Clinical Psychology Science and Practice, 24* (2), 170–185. 10.1111/cpsp.12195.

Bass, A (2003). "E" Enactments in psychoanalysis: Another medium, another message. *Psychoanalytic Dialogues, 13* (5), 657–675. 10.1080//10481881309348762

Bloom, SL, (1999). Trauma theory abbreviated. *Final Action Plan: A Coordinated Community Response to Family Violence.* Office of the Attorney General, Commonwealth of Pennsylvania.

Bromberg, PM (1993). Shadow and substance: A relational perspective on Clinical Process. *Psychoanalytic Psychology, 10* (2), 147–168. 10.1037/h0079464.

Bromberg, PM (1994). "Speak! That I may see you:" Some reflections on dissociation, reality, and analytic listening. *Psychoanalytic Dialogues, 4* (4), 517–547. 10.1080/10481889409539037.

Bromberg, PM (1998). *Standing in the Spaces.* The Analytic Press.

Bromberg, PM (2003). Something this way comes: Trauma, dissociation, and conflict: The space where psychoanalysis, cognitive science, and neuroscience overlap. *Psychoanalytic Psychology, 20* (3), 558–574. 10.1037/0736-9735.20.3.558

Chefetz, R & Bromberg, P (2004). Talking with "me" and "not-me": A dialogue. *Contemporary Psychoanlaysis, 40* (3) 409–464. 10.1080/00107530.2004.10745840.

Gillespie, A (2005). G.H. Mead: Theorist of the social act. *Journal for the Theory of Social Behaviour, 35* (1), 19–39. 10.1111/j.0021-8308.2005.00262.x

Grotstein, JS (2000). *Who is the Dreamer Who Dreams the Dream?* Analytic Press.

Hermans, HJM (2001). The dialogical self: Towards a theory of personal and cultural positioning. *Culture & Psychology, 7* (3), 243–281. 10.1177/1354067X0173001

Hermans, HJM, & Kempen, HJG (1993). *The dialogical self: Meaning as movement.* Academic Press.

Hesse, H (1929). *Steppenwolf.* (B Creighton, Trans.) Henry Holt and Company.

James, W (1890/1950). *Principles of psychology: Volumes I & II.* Dover Publications.

Janet, P (1888). *L'Automatisme psychologique: Essai de psychologie expérimentale sur les formes inférieures de l'activité humaine.* Paris: Alcan.

Kessler, RC, McLaughlin, KA, Green, JG, Gruber, MJ, Sampson, NA, Zaslavsky, AM, et al. (2010). Childhood adversities and adult psychopathology in the WHO world mental health surveys. *British Journal of Psychiatry, 197* (5), 378–385. 10.1192/bjp.bp.110.080499.

Kluft, RP (1985). Childhood multiple personality disorder: Predictors, clinical findings, and treatment results. In RP Kluft (Ed.), *Childhood antecedents of multiple personality* (pp. 167–196). American Psychiatric Press.

Kluft, RP (1991). Clinical presentations of multiple personality disorder. *Psychiatric Clinics of North America, 14*(3), 605–629. 10.1016/S0193-953X(18)30291-0.

Levenson, EA (1983/2005). The fallacy of understanding/The ambiguity of change. The Analytic Press.

Marková, I (2003a). *Dialogicality and social representations*. Cambridge University Press.

Marková, I (2003b). Constitution of the self: Intersubjectivity and dialogicality. *Culture & Psychology, 9* (3), 249–259. 10.1177/1354067X030093006

Mead, GH (1967). *Mind, self and society: From the standpoint of a social behaviorist* (Vol 1). University of Chicago Press.

Polychronis, P (2018). Integrated care, shared electronic records and the psychology profession: A cautionary tale for counseling centers. *Journal of College Student Psychotherapy, 34* (1), 1–23. 10.1080/87568225.2018.14 89745.

Rosenbaum, PJ & Webb, RE (2019). Treating trauma in the fishbowl of university and college counseling centers. *Journal of College Student Psychotherapy*. Advance online publication. 10.1080/87568225.2019.1 671293

Saunders, BE, & Adams, ZW (2014). Epidemiology of traumatic experiences in childhood. *Child and Adolescent Psychiatric Clinics of North America, 23* (2), 167–184. 10.1016/j.chc.2013.12.003.

Slochower, J (2004). *Holding and Psychoanalysis: A Relational Approach*. Routledge Publications.

Stein, A (2001). Murder and Memory. *Contemporary Psychoanalysis, 37* (7), 443–451. 10.1080.00107530.2001.10747089.

Steinbeck, J (1992). *East of Eden*. Penguin Books. (Original work published 1952).

Stern, DB (2004). The eye sees itself: Dissociation enactment and the achievement of conflict. *Contemporary Psychoanalysis, 40* (2), 197–237. 10.1080/00107530.2004.10745828

Stern, DB (2006). Opening what has been closed, relaxing what has been clenched: Dissociation and enactment over time in committed relationships. *Psychoanalytic Dialogues, 16* (6), 747–761. 10.1080/1048188070135 7446

Stern, DB (2009). *Partners in Thought: Working with Unformulated Experience, Dissociation and Enactment*. Routledge Publications.

Stern, DB (2015). *Relational Freedom: Emergent Properties of the Interpersonal Fields*. Routledge Publications.

Stern (2018). *The Infinity of the Unsaid: Unformulated Experience, Language and the Nonverbal*. Routledge Publications.

Sullivan, H (1950). The illusion of personal individuality. *Psychiatry, 13* (3), 317–332. 10.1080/00332747.1950.11022783

Sullivan, HSS (1953). *The Interpersonal Theory of Psychiatry*. New York, NY: W.W. Norton Publications.

Sullivan, HS (1956). *Clinical Studies in Psychiatry*. W. W. Norton.

van der Kolk, BA (1989). The compulsion to repeat the trauma, Reenactment, revictimization, and masochism. *Psychiatric Clinics of North America, 12* (2), 389–411. 10.1016/s0193-953x(18)30439-8.

Vygotsky, LS (1978). *Mind in Society*. Harvard University Press.

Webb, RE & Widseth, JC (2009). Traumas with and without a sense of agency. *Journal of Aggression, Maltreatment & Trauma, 18* (5), 532–546. 10.1080/10926770903050993

Yeats, WB (1932). *Words for music perhaps and other poems*. The Cuala Press.

Zittoun, T & Gillespie, A (2015). Internalization: How culture becomes mind. *Culture & Psychology, 21* (4), 477–491. 10.1177/1354067x15615809.

Chapter 7

The Complexities of Otherness[1]

Post-secondary education in the United States is often at the center of passionate discussions about dimensions of otherness. Whether pertaining to differences pertinent to race, sex, gender, religion, class, culture or differences in neurological or a host of functional body capabilities, university-aged students are frequently on the front lines of protests demanding change. The ways community members of our post-secondary institutions engage these issues often play out in powerful and complicated ways. This makes sense because education, especially at the university level, entails the development of critical thinking that often involves challenging conventional understandings of truth and right and wrong. In tandem and support of this, our institutions provide important space, both psychological and physical, for students to explore and try on new identities.

While discussions about otherness and the policies that pertain to it frequently occur between different student groups, in this chapter we focus on prototypical conversations that occur between administrators/faculty and student groups. Frequently staff (especially directors) of counseling centers are asked to offer consultation to the various constituencies. In this chapter, we offer composite examples that draw on our own experience with this. In doing so, we hope to shed light not only on the psychological processes that underlie these conversations but also on how they may occur when there are clear differences and power discrepancies.

While we think similar dynamics may be observed if we compared different groups of students, highlighting student-administrator interactions helps to show how these processes play out when one

DOI: 10.4324/9781003246558-8

group (administrators) are more secure in their position of power and privilege than others (students). It is precisely because of this discrepancy that theories that help us better understand how we relate to self and other are necessary.

We propose that an important avenue for "better understanding" comes when we map how the discussions and conflicts around sameness and otherness reflect the occupation of particular existential-relational positions. The reader will recall that in Chapter 2 we describe a developmental model that considers how our relational world expands in a linear but non-stable way from primary enmeshment with our caregiver to a fuller embrace of otherness. This process can be broken into four different developmental positions that in part address how we experience the agency and authority that is so key to our embrace of both the otherness of others and our otherness to ourselves. In this chapter, we map the discussions and conflicts around sameness and otherness that take place at our institutes onto these developmental processes. With these developmental processes in mind, we, then, offer some thoughts about how we can do better.[2]

Some important caveats

We do not think that it is necessarily the work of those calling for change to consider the developmental location of those they are asking to change. They do enough work. Nevertheless, we see our clinical focus on tolerating ambiguity and the paradoxes of living as one relevant to all of us at all times. Accordingly, our hope in this chapter is that by describing the psychological developmental processes that we see as leading to frustrating interactions around difference and change we can open up pathways for a more open embrace of otherness.

Simultaneously, we find value in extending the psychoanalytic model of development toward the level of relating between administrators and students. While there is some precedent about how psychodynamic ideas may be applied in more consultative fashion (Aron, 2012), it is an area that remains underdeveloped, especially within institutes of higher learning. Notably, while we locate some of the challenges and complexities in these situations in feelings that may have first arisen in our childhood, we do so with an eye not to shift responsibility toward how they are being played out in the here-and-now or to view one side as "adults" and the other as "children" but rather to understand more fully, so as to create the best opportunities for growth and change. In this, we recognize that the psychological underpinnings we describe below are similar in many ways for both students and administrators.

Navigating our psychological need/defense of "splitting"

Although we have described the movement between different developmental chapters elsewhere, it is necessary to begin discussing the psychological processes at play by first elaborating some of what occurs when moving between the paranoid-schizoid and depressive positions. Specifically, we have to discuss the dual processes of "splitting" and "projection." These are both some of our most fundamental psychological organizing mechanisms and also some of our most basic defenses.

Splitting and projection are the psychological hallmarks of the paranoid-schizoid position (Klein, 1975a, 1975b). Our ability to develop toward the depressive position is contingent upon the fate of these defenses. How our caregivers handle our normative needs to split and project sets the stage for our ability to move into the depressive position not only as children but also throughout life. This speaks to the ways that we are always moving between positions depending upon context and situation. When fortunate and raised in "good enough" circumstance, we are more able to move flexibly between these positions and so not remain "stuck."

Splitting and projection

Splitting originates in the baby's earliest encounter with otherness and difference. When faced with the potentially threatening discontinuity of experience, whereby their caretaker fails to meet their needs, the infant reacts by beginning to organize their world into categories of "good" and "bad" (Klein, 1975a, 1975b). Good entails experiences and conduct that help get their needs met and create feelings of security; whereas bad encompasses those experiences that lead to frustration and feelings of insecurity (Sullivan, 1953). While simplistic these categories organize the world into more stable patterns creating both experiences of continuity and sameness that lead to security.

An important part of what maintains this stability is the way that experiences that may cause upset or feelings of being "bad" can be projected unconsciously out of "me" and into "not-me." When we are babies, this "not-me" is often our primary caregiver and sometimes, it is only a "part" of them. Thus, psychodynamic clinicians such as Melanie Klein (1975a, 1975b) suggest that the "breast" becomes "bad" due to the baby not being able to get milk from it. The projection of "badness" into mother's breast is important in that it maintains the feelings that the infant themselves is "good" as is "mother" as a whole. Only a part of them is "bad." This preserves the possibility of a relationship between the baby and the good mother. In this regard, projection begins first as a way of maintaining our relational ties so that we can have our basic needs met.

Notably, the important "others" such as our caretakers have to manage the projection into them of being "bad." This process is often referred to as "metabolizing" whereby the caretaker can take the babies "projections" not as "personal attack" but rather as expressions of self-concern about both the baby's and mother's relational continuance (Allen et al., 2008). We discuss the need for mother to be able to successfully do this more extensively in Chapter 4, as part of this process importantly entails the failure of the caregiver in sustaining this process. However, when parents are "good enough," they begin to help us as babies to integrate our experiences of "good and bad" into a more cohesive whole, such that we come to learn that all people are composed of "good" and "bad" parts.

This is akin to moving from object relating to object usage. When successful, we can move from the paranoid-schizoid position of categorical organization toward more nuanced and complex views of me and you. Here, there may be an "I" (who is both good and bad) and "you" (also good and bad).

Three relational challenges of the paranoid-schizoid position

As babies develop through infancy and into toddlers and small children, they have to begin managing their own anxieties that come from projecting their badness into other people as well as the experiences whereby the parent cannot metabolize these feelings at all times. Given the nature of the projections, children have to deal with paranoid and persecutory anxieties about how the other will handle them. Note that we are not saying children are paranoid in a diagnostic sense but rather have to tolerate deep fear around the negotiation of split-off aggression and badness. In speaking of these dynamics, the psychoanalyst Jessica Benjamin (2004) coined the expressions of "doer" and "done-to" that highlight what can happen in the parent-child dynamic. There are three specific relational challenges that may emerge while navigating splitting and projection that are of note here.

Fearing retaliation from the parent: Being the "done-to"

In the first, in response to their aggression the child fears retaliation by the parent. This happens when the parent rejects the child's projections instead of taking them in and metabolizing so that they can give them back to the child in a more worked through form. Thus, for example, in response to the child's angry projections about not having a need met the parent retaliates by yelling back at the child that they are "impossible." Here, the parent does not metabolize and say something like "I know you're hungry and it's hard to be patient" but rather retaliates with their own aggression. This in turn leaves the child feeling "bad" and also victimized as the "done-to."

In their badness, the child also feels wounded by the parent, with whom the child might no longer feel safe. If this happens enough times, then, the child, in an effort to reconnect may attempt the impossible: the repudiation of separation or an effort to stitch up the wound. This results in an effort to appease their parent for whom their needs were forcing a separation in order to reassert sameness (lack of difference). In other words, the child makes an appeal to the "good" self of their M-other by being perfectly "good" themselves. This often entails an over-sensitivity to the hurt felt by the M-other (i.e., nascent others) and the child may become stuck within a mantra of "I must not cause hurt again."

This may cause the child to view their assertion as dangerous. In the move toward the depressive position, the child may become overwhelmed with feelings of guilt and shame at having hurt their loved parent. Moreover, their own sense of "goodness" becomes performative and maybe even fake, an "as if" (Sullivan, 1953). It is born out of a need to smooth over and mollify, and it is not genuinely felt or earned. This gives it a certain fragility and instability.

Our experience of ourselves as "perpetrator" or "doer"

In the second relational challenge, the child experiences themselves not as the victim but as the perpetrator of the hurt and comes to experience themselves as the aggressor. Thus, when the parent yells at the child that they are "impossible," the child does not feel victimized by the parent but rather identifies as the "aggressor." Here, the child worries that their aggression has "killed" their parent. Often what differentiates the child's experience of being the "doer" and not the "done to" resides in the parent's response. If the parent "disappears" such that the child's needs go unmet, then they are likely to identify as a "murderer."

Notably, sometimes when parents who are killed off come back, it is often with a certain overcompensation. So, in the face of aggression, they might withdraw before then coming back to the relationship with the child with "abundance" as a way of trying to re-establish it. From the child's perspective, then, rage leads to disappearance and then a confusing feeling of the parent trying to "make it up" to them. The child may then come to learn that their aggression generates an emotional response of care that eventually facilitates attention.

The mantra becomes: "I hurt in order to get care and attention."

Our need to harden and numb ourselves to the other

Finally, a third dynamic may emerge where the child, being overwhelmed by experiences of hurting and repairing, seeks to harden their sensitivity to the hurt, both the M-other's and their own. Here, then, there is a practiced (even if not always conscious) insensitivity to the hurt of M-other and a mantra of "I'm not hurt, because hurt does not exist for me" (or by extension, for others).

Notably, these reactions can be discrete and unique but also combined in such a way that parent and child engage in some combination of all forms of relating. This generates a confusing mix of what to expect and an inability to establish a stable pattern. The lack of stability can create very destabilizing and disorienting feelings of chaos on the part of the child who becomes "mystified" (Levenson, 1989) at what the parent expects and what is needed to be secure.

The depressive position

When we and our caregivers can successfully navigate our paranoid-schizoid anxieties emergent around difference, we move into the depressive position where we begin to see "good" and "bad" as residing in each of us. Then, we have to be concerned with how our aggressive strivings to differentiate has harmed the other (hence, Winnicott's reference to this as the period of "concern"). We often experience guilt at having harmed the other, which leads to efforts at making reparations. This is an important process of building a secure sense of self. Our sturdiness involves integrating our capacity to harm with the possibilities of repair as a human endeavor. In this, we may become depressed at our inability to satisfy fully the needs of the other and so mourn our incompleteness. With this comes the opportunity for grace as we realize our shared humanity and begin to embody curiosity about other ways of being. Once we can feel secure in ourselves and the world we occupy, we can feel safe in learning about other ways of being.

It is, however, quite rare that any of us emerge out of this developmental period fully consolidated and unshakeably secure. We tend to be a mix of conflicting feelings that result from our existential situation and so we may move back toward a more paranoid-schizoid position if threatened or anxious. This move back toward the paranoid-schizoid position is often highlighted by the earlier need to preserve our view of ourselves as "good." Accordingly, we return to our defenses of splitting and projection. Thus, when challenged with views of ourselves that seem threatening, we may split off our badness such that we are "good" and those challenging us are "bad." Or, anticipating being challenged, we may act in ways that ensure our "goodness" by learning the correct terms and words so as to not offend, even though in doing so we come across as inauthentic. Still, in other cases, we may withdraw into ourselves so as to not be threatened and disturbed.

Dealing with otherness in the context of higher education

Rather than view the above relational challenges as pathological, from a developmental perspective we recognize that the ways we meet them are necessary to ensure that our needs are met sufficiently for us to survive. Moreover, this perspective helps us to think about what may be at stake in moments and conversations that generate anxiety about our presence and ongoingness. This is especially true within the contexts of higher education where there are spaces intentionally carved out for thinking about otherness and difference.

For example, discussions of "white guilt," defined as the feelings of individual and collective guilt that some of us white people may feel for harm resulting from intentional or unintentional racist treatment of ethnic minorities, are common in today's higher education climate (DiAngelo, 2018). From our perspective, what is sometimes so difficult for White people to bear and experience in these discussions is not only the "guilt about hurting a racialized other" but also the way that this guilt may echo about the earlier hurts we have caused others, especially our primary caregiver. As a result, when confronted with how we are currently causing harm, despite our best intentions, we react not only in the here and now but with all of our history of causing harm.

As Kendi (2019) notes, our racist attitudes and actions not only are hard to bear because of the pain they cause but also due to our feeling that these actions make us "bad" people. Note in this the recourse to earlier feelings of guilt and badness and their echoes of the paranoid-schizoid position. This generates not only anxiety of harming the other but also worry about the retaliation and loss of esteem that may come from our actions. This threatens our feeling of "goodness" and so threatens to overwhelm us with a sense that we are fundamentally a "bad person."

Once we are grappling with the issue of our "goodness and badness," it can be difficult to find solid footing so that we can reflect on our actions in a way that leads to growth. We may be required to understand our harmful action not only as it has occurred presently but also need to acknowledge our historic anxiety around hurting. It is necessary to find our footing in this regard because moving beyond the hurt requires *meaningful* actions as the substance for creating repair.

The need for meaningful action and the role of campus leaders

If we continue with the above example, while white students may feel "guilt" and anxiety, students of color may then be left to grapple with their own feelings of possibly having caused this "hurt." There are also frustrations for students of color about white students not "getting it" that comes with feeling a need to defend their existence. There can be resentment and anger about having to "teach" others with a commensurate wish that white students would do their own homework about their effect on the others who are other. That these feelings make sense and are entirely appropriate given the structural racism we are socialized into does not make bearing them easier.

It is here that we see the crucial role of campus leaders who serve as "leading parts" in the community system (Bertalanffy, 1968). Specifically, our leaders, especially in our administrations (and so including us), have to be the ones to take on these dilemmas not in a removed fashion but directly and meaningfully. We must not fall into the paranoid-schizoid position where we rely on projection or avoidance. If we do, we must work our way out of this position as best we can. Simultaneously, we must not become so subsumed by the anxiety about our own "badness" that we seek quickly to plaster over wounds that cannot be dressed without a thorough examination. We must accept that real repair is difficult and even sometimes simply not possible.

Toward this end, we need to embody leadership which understands that in our efforts to regain our lost hold on the depressive position we must move with care and concern for all parties. In this, we have to be able to tolerate the "badness" that may come from recognizing the limits of repair. We must be able to engage recognition that needs will be frustrated. It is in our response to these complex demands that we think we help enable the college and university system to move beyond the "doer done-to" dynamic that Jessica Benjamin (2004) describes.

In this we might think that our campus leaders can hold the tension between A <> Non-A such that new meanings may emerge in how we relate to self and other. It is within the experience of intense affects, including anger, shame and guilt that the relational field may collapse such that we become fixated upon a singular point or feeling. Then, we know what we are "bad" and what the other is "good." From this position, new development that allows for a broader and fuller recognition is difficult if not impossible. Keeping the space open for elaboration involves a willingness to sit with the tension of not knowing such that new meanings can emerge.

Paying attention to the ongoing developmental dynamics hopefully helps ourselves and our leaders recognize the complexities at play and provides some guidance on thinking when these complicated questions emerge. In considering these situations, we are not saying that adolescent students or adult administrators are "acting like children" or "being childish" when issues arise or passions are inflamed. Rather, we see these moments as occurring with real and present hurts, pains and age. However, we also think that working through them in a way that moves past appeasement and mollification requires the consideration of how our childhood developmental challenges and issues can weave into the mix and be relevant to current negotiations.

Typical administrator situations

At an administrative level, perhaps the most typical situation occurs when students express criticism of a specific administrator who is associated with a policy or action with which they take issue. Some recent examples are around "trigger warnings," academic honesty, the school's investments or questions of divestments, a stance toward social justice, a recent hiring, how the school adjudicates issues of sexual assault and discrimination and so forth.[3]

If we, as this administrator, operate from a history where the prevailing feeling is "I must not hurt again," there is a risk that our decision around the issue will be made to appease the students rather than engage them. When we lead with our wishes to be experienced as the good loving one who does not hurt or cause pain, there can be little tolerance for making decisions, which do not support our effort to feel loved, by others. We pale at the task of making an unpopular decision because we have organized our world dichotomously. Hence, if we are not being experienced as "good," then we fear by default that we are the "bad" parent who is insufficient and wounding. Thus, we struggle to say "no" or to define a position to which others can push back.

Even if we are generally supportive of the student issue, if it is made with an eye toward getting back in good graces rather than embrace the whole of the student and the issue, we are not authentically and fully engaging with them. For instance, we might not be holding space for critical thinking of the issue and exploring the nuances of it but rather rushing to fix things. While we may be accused, perhaps even correctly, in asserting privilege in exerting nuance and thought, it is often also within the purview of educational institutions. If done with an eye toward embrace and understanding and not avoidance, it allows for the type of engagement that we think moves beyond doer and done to. Without engaging fully, we attempt to circumvent the students' developmental need to "cut out" and highlight difference. In striving to highlight difference, the student may locate the administrator as "other" regardless of how we personally view ourselves.

This "cutting out," whether reality based[4] or not, feels like an indictment of our wounding ways and an exposure of our shortcomings or ways that are disappointing. Here, we are often surprised that our "goodness" has not been seen, and we experience students' developmental needs to define and oppose as a personal attack. This drives up our anxiety and threatens to move us from a more open relational perspective to a closed one of being either "good" or "bad." In our concern with being "good," we can easily falter in our capacity to react from a balanced perspective.

Complicating things further is when students emerge with an issue that challenges the community and generates a bewildering back and forth amongst us administrators who are empowered to make a decision about the issue. This is akin to parents at home not being on the same page (one parent says "no," the other says "yes"). There are at times indulgent "yes's" stemming from our unconscious effort to "stitch up the gap" in the cut of difference and return the identity-seeking students to our fold where we are the good loving parent. There also, however, can be strident "no's" which come out in the wake of us feeling frustrated by students' developmental needs and the sense that nothing we offer will be enough, so "Why keep offering?"

What is lacking in both these reactions is a more thoughtful, slowed down and measured response where we articulate differences, explore rationales, and work on a negotiated response with the students which is not so powerfully driven by our own developmental anxieties. The anxious, knee-jerk and inconsistent response does not give the students sturdy difference to better find their own separate feet and, thereby, to feel that their concerns are being taken in earnest. There is then pain on both ends. From our administrative perspective, there is the threat of the woeful drop into again being the "bad one" and from the student's perspective there is the disappointment in having insufficient opportunity to herald their separateness.

Sometimes in these situations, our reactive "no" prompts students to seek counsel and support of other administrators or faculty, some who may deal with these issues less frequently. Not only might these administrators fall into redoing the dynamic, but now, when contrasted with us as the unsympathetic and "bad" administrator, may face even more pressure to assert a "yes." In other words, the students seek to find others who are empowered administratively who will see in responding to the initial administrative "no" the opportunity to be the voice of "yes." We, as this other administrator, too frequently hope our "yes" will make us, especially by contrast with our colleague, the long last good guy we have wanted to be in order to deny our own wounding past.

We should add here that over time there is the potential for cynicism to take hold within both students and us as administrators. Students' experiences are limited by their time within the community, even if there is the possibility of the kind of limited but lifelong engagement that being an alumnus allows. This time-limited experience as an actual student perhaps protects students from too quickly falling into a cynical perspective. We administrators, however, are often in place for long tenures, and, therefore, this resort to cynicism, under the ravages of time, can especially be a danger to us.

Much like when parenting young children whose needs are overwhelming; we may feel like nothing we do is "good enough" and that students are going to be "unhappy with us no matter what." This may derive not out of actual thoughtful and soulful engagement with our students but instead out of the frustration of having offered "yes's" to appease, "yes's" which fail to quiet down the student needs. This speaks to the mis-attunement that exists when operating

from a position of "good" and "bad," and it is a feeling and perspective that might very well be central in characterizations of the
current generation as entitled.

The potential for this level of functioning is the black hole of
gravity for nearly all communities, and it is, unfortunately, the most
typical position where most groups function, especially when they
expand out beyond the dyadic interpersonal into "large-group"
psychology (Volkan, 2013). Communities are in a constant effort to
forbear from being drawn down into this position, drawn down into
finding their togetherness or collective "good-me-ness" by appointing
divergent others, both within and without their community, as the
"bad-me's" that must be begrudgingly tolerated if not rejected all
together.

Typical student situation

As we proceed to look at the situation more from the student's
perspective, we must caution against the danger of simply flipping
what might seem like some needle of blame in the other direction.
There are notable power differentials between students and administrators not to mention the developmental slant we have been describing throughout. In response to the attempts by key "leading
parts" of the community to stitch up the gap in the "cut out" by
seeking commonality and sameness, students might rightfully feel
unheard and unseen. Comments by we administrators, such as "we
are all on the same page" or "we are all in agreement and are one,"
are essential attempts at mollifying the student need for recognition, a
type of recognition which we feel comes first through an acknowledgment of difference and then a willingness on the part of we administrators (and at times by students not in the fray) to hold this
difference, even if it feels unfair to us.

When, instead, we try to be the reassuring non-wounding good
parent-administrator, student leaders, in order to be seen as a distinguishable other, have to push harder. In an ironic way, efforts at
too quickly stitching the gap feel worse because the meaningful dialogue that students crave is foreclosed. This is further complicated
when students and student leaders pivot from significant histories,
where surviving the "cut out" of separation and difference from their

primary caregivers and peers has required them to protect themselves from their anxieties about having wounded M-other. In these cases, students anticipate the other to be hurt and/or hurtful and therefore act to protect themselves in advance with a hardened stance, which limits the patience required of them in order to weather the challenging conversation about difference which needs to occur.

When this situation lasts long enough, we administrators often become cynical, skeptical and even forlorn. Students, if they do not succumb fully to hopelessness and despair, are often mobilized into an angry agitation. Much like when children realize that their parent will not meet their needs, students feel that they are negotiating with immovable others. We know that this is a terrible situation because students will turn away from us as administrators and from other institutional supports in order to "do it themselves." For these students, trying to stitch up the gap of difference and separation comes from a history where doing so is tantamount to the loss of self. In the recrudescence of this during their life on campus, there is a history-fueled determination, in essence, to fight tooth and nail the threat to their sense of identity. This is so because the realm of "being" is confined either to existing as "other" or as the ongoing completion of the societal "M-other."

In these cases, relationships between students and administrators (and sometimes also other students) feel destined toward a perfect storm of conflict. On the one hand, there are we administrators who see diversity and separateness as an issue that demands acknowledgment of sameness. On the other, there are students whose adaptive histories position them to fight sameness in way which feels existential in its gravity. Proclaiming their diverseness/difference and encouraging others to do the same means not stitching up the gap but instead spreading it further apart. At this point, community negotiations and conversation can easily descend into the binary of "good" and "bad," a "us" versus "them" dynamic.

Ironically, in some extreme cases, this effort often entails energized demand that others define their otherness, often out of the fearful concern that true safety and understanding can only be found in the sameness of difference. Then there might be a tendency to see people as means to an end. Failure to achieve a goal may lead to a rejection of the other as a whole.

How do we do better?

There are, of course, many ways to do better at diversifying our communities and, thereby, benefit from the enrichment that comes from this. Others (Helling & Chandler, 2019) have elaborated ideas about how this can be done. Much of what has been proposed has been stated and restated. We will not repeat these ideas in any detail, but in essence they include embracing diversity by a plethora of efforts that range from the straightforward: work diligently to increase the actual numbers of those in the community who are "different," to the more challenging: develop support structures that reflect appreciation of the history, culture, and sensitivities of the "different others" that are invited into the community. Such support structures encompass everything from creating new academic courses through offering "sensitivity" trainings through building physical spaces that are welcoming.

As all of us in the field at ground level know, implementing these ideas, unfortunately, is more often easier said than done. Hence, we recognize that as we join the chorus of those who echo these ideas, we also join the throng that continues to fall short. The idea, however, of falling short is in some ways a key notion in this chapter. In fact, it is in a focused deliberation of one aspect of how we fall short that we think this chapter offers a perspective that is not commonly weaved into the mix of ideas about "how we can do better."

We take for granted that we are historical beings but seldom do we take this sufficiently seriously to keep it consciously present as a factor in how we experience ourselves in relation to others in the present time. We propose that better understanding of the developmental sequence that pertains to the embrace our own and other's differentness is of fundamental utility for doing better. Especially within communities of higher education where intellectual perspective is heralded as important for informing our view of the world, ourselves, and those around us, it makes good sense to consider how our own individual histories with separation and difference might map onto to what we know about the common, developmental sequence relevant to this. Knowing where our feet stand not only in relation to our own individual journey but also in terms of the trek common to all is important for truly knowing where we tend to function in relation to others and in relation to ourselves. And this, we propose, is of key importance for being able to implement the ideas we note above that are more commonly associated with doing better with diversity.

With the anchoring understanding of developmental positions and with courage to consider how our personal histories weave in and through these positions, we propose that we better fortify ourselves as an administrator or faculty member to remain able to listen carefully and astutely when we are told by an upset student: "You don't get it. You don't know what it's like to be me (or us). You're insensitive." While, indeed, we might be in that moment exactly what the student is accusing us of, with an anchoring understanding of developmental positions we, at least, have the opportunity to check our perspective. We have the opportunity, for instance, *maybe* to not take the student's comment as an insightful indictment of our "bad me" who damaged our M-other with the way we "cut out" our being from his or hers. We have the opportunity to keep our reaction in the present. We are more able *not* to speak and react to the student from a historical subtext which might incline us to undo our sense of being destructive with either compliant agreeableness which implicitly pleads for favorable reappraisal of us as a "good guy" or with puffed up toughness which implicitly accuses the student of arrogant entitlement. Instead, we are *maybe* more able to stay fully present in the prevailing context and to keep conversational space available for the thoughtful reflection and exploration that the comment deserves. A true embrace of difference and diversity demands nothing less.

Accordingly, we think it is important that our institutions make a concerted effort to incorporate developmental ideas of sameness and difference into our community. This kind of effort should be community-wide. For students, it might most propitiously be done during orientation activities for first-year students and through outreach activities throughout the year. The emphasis would be on understanding the psychological processes of attachment, separation, and relating to self and other, a version of which we have shared in this chapter. Anecdotally, we think that desire to learn more about these processes is why groups with the title of "relating to self and other" or "connecting with self and other" are so popular at institutions. It's not just that people yearn to connect to other people but that they also want to learn how these processes occur.

One way to accomplish this is to offer community members, especially students (but certainly not just limited to them) programs and workshops designed to share information about their world views and backgrounds. Hearing and sharing personal stories helps us recognize what is the same between us but also what is different. Being able to recognize the universality of comparing sameness to difference not only helps us appreciate what is different about ourselves and others but also what may be different and even contradictory within ourselves.

Conclusion

In the face of the powerful prevailing and countervailing psychological winds in the chaos of our own inner worlds, the simplicity of a binary solution is enormously appealing. Thinking in terms of "good" and "bad" and right and wrong should be treated suspiciously. While it is a natural stage of relating during development, it enforces demands upon self and other and leads to circular reenactments which limit fuller engagement with self and other.

Doing better means embracing complexity with a humility we hope that recognizes the possibility of finding ourselves not only in relationship with others but also within others. As we end, we are reminded of the words of the psychoanalyst D.W. Winnicott (1960) that there is no baby without a mother; no mother without a baby. Similarly, there is no college without students and students without the college. It is only when we share in the struggle of wrestling with our sameness and difference from self and other that we are able to hope to adequately advance ahead.

Notes

1 A version of this chapter was published as Webb, R.E. & Rosenbaum, P. (2021). Embracing diversity: The complexities of reckoning and accepting otherness. *Integrative Psychological and Behavioral Science, 50*(1), 30–46. DOI: 10.1007/s12124-020-09582-9.

2 We realize that our aim here is quite ambitious. However, we consider the theory that we offer and its application to be an important foundational perspective that

respects the complexity entailed in any attempt at addressing the phenomena of relating to self and other, especially in the arena of group functioning. As Francisco González says, there is a need within the "Relational tradition" of psychoanalysis to address more fully "work with primitive states" and "groupal object relations – that is, one-to-many identifications or the individually held, "we"-part of subjectivity (2016, p. 524). Hence, as the increasingly intolerance of otherness drives so much current unrest in the United States and seems to underlie emergent human rights offenses, we think the ambition of our aim is a necessary risk even if we do not think we have a tonic, per se, for the intolerance. In demonstrating the ways, psychological theories of development inform how we work as consultants to the college around particularly thorny issues we hope to stir consideration that the value of this type of thinking and approach might also have wider application.

3 It is worth noting that both authors either have been or are college administrators and so the pull toward operating from this position is understood personally.

4 Again, one might argue that knowing about various aspects of identity, culture and background is a reasonable expectation and that our description comes out of a place of privileging our identities. To a certain extent this feels true it is an onus on administrators to be as educated as possible. But more than education, we think the attitudes of openness and curiosity are what allows for true tolerance and acceptance and as we are arguing this only comes out of a developmental process where one can tolerate imperfections in self and other.

References

Allen, JG, Fonagy, P, & Batement, AW (2008). *Mentalizing in clinical practice*. American Psychiatric Publishing, Inc.

Aron, L (2012). Psychoanalysis in the workplace: An introduction. *Psychoanalytic Dialogues, 22* (5), 511–516. 10.1080/10481885.2012.717041.

Benjamin, J (2004). Beyond does and done to: An intersubjective view of third ness. *The Psychoanalytic Quarterly, 73* (1), 5–46. 10.1002/j.2167-4086.2004.tb0015.x

Bertalanffy, L. von (1968). *General system theory: Foundations, development, applications*. George Braziller.

DiAngelo, R (2018). *White fragility: Why it's so hard for white people to talk about racism*. Beacon Press.

Gonzalez, F (2016). On the relation to non-relationality. *Psychoanalytic Dialogues, 26* (5), 522–531. 10.1080/10481889909539308.

Helling, J & Chandler, GE (2019). Meeting the psychological health & growth needs of black college students: Culture, resonance and resilience. *Journal of College Student Psychotherapy*. Advance online publication. 10.87568225.2019.1660291

Kendi, IX (2019). *How to be an antiracist*. One World.

Klein, M (1975a). *The collected works of Melanie Klein, Volume I, love, guilt and reparation and other works 1921–1945*. The Free Press.

Klein, M (1975b). *The collected works of Melanie Klein, Volume III, envy, gratitude and other works 1946–1963*. The Free Press.

Levenson, EA (1989). Whatever happened to the cat? – Interpersonal perspectives on the self. *Contemporary Psychoanalysis*, *25*, 537–553.

Sullivan, HSS (1953). *The interpersonal theory of psychiatry*. W.W. Norton.

Volkan, V (2013). Large-group-psychology in its own right: Large-Group identity and peace-making. *International Journal of Applied Psychoanalytic Studies*, *10* (3), 210–246. DOI: 10.1002/aps.1368

Winnicott, DW (1960). The theory of the parent-infant relationship. In D Winnicott (Ed.), *The maturational processes and the facilitating environment* (pp. 37–45). Routledge. 10.4324/9780429482410-3

Chapter 8

A Macro-perspective on Groups and Group Identification [1]

Our earlier chapters have focused largely on how an understanding of the four existential-relational positions informs our thinking about individual development. In this last chapter, we will "zoom out" and consider the relevance of these positions for understanding functioning at a larger scale, how these positions speak to affiliation with tribes or groups. We draw inspiration from George Orwell (1945) and so think of these tribes as "nationalism," "patriotism" and "internationalism." In this, we think our effort is consistent with what Francisco González recently described as a need within the "Relational tradition" of psychoanalysis to address more fully "work with primitive states" and "groupal object relations – that is, one-to-many identifications or the individually held, 'we'-part of subjectivity" (2016, p. 524).

Although our consideration of tribalism is relevant beyond the margins of late adolescence and young adulthood, we think it is especially pertinent to college-aged students. Generally speaking, this period of time is when students of traditional college age blossom into awareness of political and moral issues. With this awareness and emerging perspective is often a deep passion that leads to energetic involvement in political activism and group affiliations.

We who are faculty, staff and administrators often are engaged intimately with the community dynamics that attend to this, and we can be challenged to find an anchoring perspective. Lastly, although each generation might think that the issues they confront are unique, there can be little argument that current world affairs are consumingly important. Against the backdrop of ever more manifest proof

DOI: 10.4324/9781003246558-9

that climate change is upon us in consequential ways, there is the emergence of COVID-19 with its ravaging effects on our health and economies and its far-reaching implications for what new normal(s) we face in family, social and business gatherings. Into this mix is the plethora of powerful protests about racism that have re-surfaced in our cities, along with energized counter-protests about lawlessness. In short, in the lap of all the societal chaos that we are experiencing, there is abundant reason to look for avenues that organize our perspective.

In this regard, "tribalism" is a word that has garnered both good and bad attention. We are in agreement with Clark and Winegard's (2020) argument that although tribalism evolved in the face of our long human history with intergroup competition and conflict, it is not "inherently bad" (p. 1). Nonetheless, and again in agreement with Clark and Winegard (2020), we think that membership in some tribes can "lead to ideological thinking and sacred values that distort cognitive processing of putatively objective information" (p. 1; see also Tong & von Hippel, 2020). We also note that the available data suggest that "tribalism and concomitant biases are part of human nature, and that no group, not even one's own, is immune" (Clark et al., 2019, p. 592; Ditto et al., 2018). Rudyard Kipling appreciates this when he says: "The individual has always had to struggle to keep from being overwhelmed by the tribe. To be your own man [sic] is a hard business. If you try it, you'll be lonely often, and sometimes frightened" (Gordon, 1967, p. 7).

In this chapter, we discuss several types of tribalism. We start with two types of group organization that Orwell introduces in his 1945 essay, *Notes on Nationalism,* before then introducing a third to which Orwell gives only passing mention. In this effort, we specifically examine the manners that certain developmental existential-relational positions significantly incline us toward affiliation with one of these tribal types versus another *regardless* of our particular political ideology.

We grant that starting with George Orwell might seem like an odd choice. Looking to history for precedent is always complicated because each time period has its uniqueness. Nonetheless, we can look to other times in our history with chaos; if not for solutions, then at least for perspective that might open new vistas. Writing at the end of World War II, a period which evidenced some of the most destructive effects of tribalism, Orwell grapples with the dynamics which underlie the fervor of nationalism, a perspective that contributed mightily to the rise of the second world war and which Orwell saw as persisting in new forms in the aftermath of the war.

While Orwell does not specifically use the word "tribalism," we think his contrasting descriptions of nationalism and patriotism distinguish two fundamental types of it which are useful for locating ourselves in the present time. The linking of tribalism with nationalism is something Czech philosopher, Ernest Gellner, notes: "Tribalism never prospers, for when it does, everyone will respect it as a true nationalism, and no one will dare call it tribalism" (1983/ 2006, p. 84).

What is at stake in this discussion is a question that the Black Lives Movement is currently demanding that US society address: When can our various institutions and social practices be reformed and when does change require something more than reformation? Toward this end, we consider whether certain types of tribal memberships are so harmful that they defy efforts at reform and, therefore, require a more extreme response. Accordingly, we try and trace the inter-tribe dynamics that can emerge when one group challenges another, and we consider ways that tribes defend and attack one another. We acknowledge that some existential threats require actions from within the tribe. Since the consequences of this action are often grave and destructive both on our campuses and outside of them, we take the exploration of how this comes about to be a matter for serious reflection.

George Orwell: On nationalism, patriotism and internationalism

Nationalism

Orwell describes nationalism as "the habit of identifying oneself with a single nation or other unit, placing it beyond good or evil and recognizing no other duty than that of advancing its interests" (1945/ 2018, p. 2). Within this, an assumption prevails that "human beings can be classified like insects and that whole blocks of ... people can be confidently labelled 'good' or 'bad'" (1945/2018, p. 1). Orwell adds:

"The abiding purpose of every nationalist is to secure more power and more prestige, *not* [original italics] for himself but for the…unit in which he [sic] has chosen to sink his own individuality" (1945/2018, p. 2). While Orwell here seems to have in mind the fascist regimes of Hitler, Mussolini and Franco as the expression of *nationalism* (Orwell, 1938/2010), we note that the impulse to categorize and label finds expression in numerous ways throughout our histories, including, for instance, the way slaves were degradingly classified in the United States and the way that Asian-American citizens were imprisoned in the United States during WWII. Orwell, in fact, extends his concern about nationalism to "such movements and tendencies as Communism, political Catholicism, Zionism, Antisemitism, Trotskyism and Pacifism" (1945/2018, p. 3).

Patriotism

Orwell is less expansive about patriotism, but his comments are important for registering the different levels of tribalism and for articulating different social consequences. He says,

> By 'patriotism' I mean devotion to a particular place and a particular way of life, which one believes to be the best in the world but has no wish to force on other people (1945/2018, p. 2). Orwell describes patriotism as defensive, both militarily and culturally.

Since patriotism is about ways of living, the appeals within the patriotic tribe are less about negatively categorizing others who are different and more about ensuring one's own continuance.

Thus, what differentiates patriotism and nationalism is that nationalism is outward looking and advancing, whereas patriotism is inward looking and more tolerant of difference. However, both systems function at the level of placing self and other into categories. For nationalism, this occurs within the sorting into good and bad, whereas for patriotism it entails a particular location and way of living.

Internationalism/globalism

Orwell offers only the slightest reference to what we think of as a third type of tribalism, "an internationalist outlook" (1945/2018,

p. 12). We think our focus should expand to include *globalism*. In this tribe we, as people, recognize that we live within the boundaries that delineate a nation, but that we think of those boundaries as useful for designation rather than delimitation. In other words, within an internationalist perspective, we think more of our own nation as one in a community of nations, a community that is ultimately mutually dependent for survival and well-being. Globalism is a tribe, in a sense, that seeks to subvert conventional tribalism with endorsement of the idea that "We are all in this together." However, globalism is not just tolerant of difference but seeks and respects it, understanding that difference makes life richer and more interesting. Within globalism is the possibility of belonging to more than one nation, meaning that we can be travelers and not hold loyalty to one way of being. So, the good to be pursed is the common good rather than "my nation's good."

Orwell's classification of social systems, including the internationalist one that we add, provides a lens for thinking about ways we organize ourselves. It does not, however, speak to the individual and group psychologies that prompt us to associate more with one or the other.

The role of our existential-relational positions in our tribal affiliations

To consider how we affiliate within tribes, we focus primarily upon the paranoid-schizoid and depressive positions. We note the transcendent position as important for consideration of globalism. As we hope the reader appreciates from our expositions in earlier chapters, these existential positions reflect how we emerge into the world and then engage it as an individuated self. The task of emerging as a *self* entails differentiation from others but also a progression in recognizing *others'* individuations, their *otherness* to our own sense of identity. As perhaps the reader can anticipate, finding one's own self and dealing with the otherness of those who are "not-me" is the bath of complexity in which tribalism lives. Notably, given our previous, extended discussions about the existential-relational positions, here we focus on the elements of them that are pertinent to tribalism.

Paranoid-schizoid position

Since our identity begins to emerge within the paranoid-schizoid position as a result of separation from our primary caregivers, it is also where we begin to recognize the colors of difference. At this time, however, difference still feels threatening to our emerging "me-ness" and so limits others to not being distinct, but rather people who are "not-me." This means their importance to "me" is limited to their instrumental value. As such, the otherness of others is flat and acontextual.

Depressive position

It is in our emergence toward the depressive position (Chapters 2, 3 and 4) that others begin to take shape and become "subjects." Essential to this is the recognition and experience of the emerging self that no symbiosis – no matter how desirable – is fulfilling and stable. Moving into the depressive position involves recognizing that no caregiver, no matter how extraordinarily attuned to us, can fully meet our needs.

This experience creates a disjunction which fosters frustration and anxiety in both ourselves and our caregiver which our caregivers need to manage in themselves and within us. If they can survive our upset and even embrace it with a loving understanding of why we are discombobulated, then they can emerge from being "bad" existential threats who fail us in our needs (thereby threatening our existence) to being safe. They begin to be others who we see as "you" and whose contextual experience of the world is something about which we can be curious and concerned. Thus, they take shape with dimensionality.

The transcendent position

In the *transcendent position*, we briefly note, there is a further evolution in the appreciation of difference and otherness. Hermann Hesse captures the prevailing view when he says, "Every age, every culture, every custom and tradition has its own character, its own weakness and its own strength, its beauties and ugliness" (1929/1990, p. 22). In this position, we more fully embrace the subjectivity of our selfhood and its inextricable existence within the confines of culture.

Identity is appreciated for the elements of its construction that are essentially socially determined. The relativity and ungraspable nature of truth is accepted; we come to appreciate what Jean Paul Sartre is arguing when he says: We are nothing, that "[n]othingness carries being in its heart" (1966, p. 52).

As such, we come to appreciate that otherness is not limited to others. There is otherness that is built into the dilemma of being human, and we understand that identity and being-ness is "radically dialogic" (Felman, 1987, p. 125) both for "me" and for "you." From the transcendent position that, which Herman Hesse says in his novel, *Steppenwolf*, makes good sense: "[E]very ego, so far from being a unity is in the highest degree a manifold world, a constellated heaven, a chaos of forms, of states and stages of inheritances and potentialities" (1929/1990, p. 59).

Ambivalence and fluidity

It is important, however, to realize that our emergence into separation is never something that is done without ambivalence. Hence, it is never securely held. While we develop linearly through these existential-relational positions, we are always moving between them in our everyday functioning. Under certain circumstances, especially ones which threaten our welfare, we can easily descend from a transcendental "We are all in this together...we are one tribe" to a paranoid-schizoid position where "I and mine" are all that is of importance. Interestingly, Ibram X. Kendi, author and scholar, offers an analogous appreciation of "movement" and identity in a comment about being racist or antiracist. He says, "We can be racist one minute and antiracist the next. What we say about race, what we do about race, in each moment, determines what – not who – we are" (2019, p. 10).

Returning to Orwell: The paranoid-schizoid and nationalism

Linking the paranoid-schizoid and depressive positions to Orwell's nationalism and patriotism enriches our understanding of these types of tribalism. It allows us to speculate about what makes nationalism or patriotism so appealing to us, especially as regards what purpose they serve for our state of being-ness and the demands we then make of society.

Paranoid-schizoid position and nationalism

In nationalism, for instance, we can hear that the way the world is cast in simplistic terms, "binary" terms, reflects a deep anxiety about separation and difference with a wish for the return to the imagined bliss of oneness. With appreciation of this embedded paranoid-schizoid mentality, a fair summary of Orwell's nationalism tribe is: We are good. Those who are not us are bad. Our goal is to prevail, and if we can do so, we will again be whole and happy in our one-ness. We are not interested in facts because facts require considera-tion of otherness and appreciation of context. These perspectives impede our wish for a dominance which insures us a home in which we all live as the one and only family.

Orwell appreciates the powerful allure of this existential position which within nationalism promises an approximation of fulfillment. He says,

> Nationalism is power hunger tempered by self-deception. Every nationalist is capable of the most flagrant dishonesty, but he is also – since he is conscious of serving something bigger than himself – unshakeably [sic] certain of being in the right. (1945/ 2018, p. 4)

The promise of certainty in nationalism harkens back to our fun-damental security with mother and the bliss of oneness. The com-promise of this certainty is that allegiance to nationalism prevents us from recognizing the otherness in all our fellow human beings and so limits our embrace of the full richness of the world.

The tenor of this kind of tribalism can be heard in the present political climate in the United States with the appeal to "Make American Great Again." The idea of a return to greatness can be seen as a wish for return to an imagined time of bliss, a period of oneness where there was no separation of beings and hence no experience of difference. There is no consideration of "great for whom." Similarly, there is no recognition that for many "others" it was not great at all.

When blinded by nationalism and the illusory promise of un-challenged oneness, it is, then, a logical step to seek the realization of this by building, not only metaphorically but also in actuality, bigger and stronger walls to keep out those who embody difference. There is incentive to expel or send back those who are "not us."

The push and pull dynamics of nationalism

To further flesh out our point, we need to consider some of the forces that maintain nationalism. As stated earlier, we are suggesting that there is a fundamental instability in our ability as humans to sustain our embrace of separateness from others. This stems not only from the longing we feel to rejoin the body of our mother but also the ways we develop into the larger symbolic order. Through internalizing semiotic process and structure, we inevitably also bring in many of the systematic ways that the other, regardless of the type of other (i.e., defined by race, gender, neurodiversity, sexual orientation and religion), is perceived as different and so threatening. This means that all of us as people have internalized attitudes of racism, sexism, classism, ableism, etc. (Kendi, 2019).

Our very participation in the institutions and structures that enable our abilities to navigate the world ensures this. Our various activities, practices and attitudes help us gain awareness of these biases and attitudes which in turn gives us greater ability to reckon with them. However, we are all susceptible to moving toward more harmful internalized positions, such that even as we may become more open minded in some directions, we can potentially become more closed in others. This seems so because psychoanalyst, Anthony Storr, writes,

> The majority of mankind want or need some all-embracing belief system which purports to provide an answer to life's mysteries, and are not necessarily dismayed by the discovery that their belief system, which they proclaim as 'the truth,' is incompatible with the beliefs of other people. (1996, p. 198)

One way we are able to "transcend" this longing for a return to "one-ness" as well as internalized positions, even if not in some unshakeable way, is to hold an appreciation for our fundamental incompleteness as beings. This existential reality fuels our fraternal pursuit of truth, with truth being something which always, ultimately eludes any of our grasps. As Jacques Lacan says: "It is Truth in fact which throws off the mask in his words, but only in order for the spirit to take on another and more deceiving one" (1968, p. 34); "[t]he truth … is that which runs after truth" (1978, p. 188). In other words, we huddle or dance together as beings always in a state of change, and as we march toward mortality, as psychoanalysts Wilfred Bion (1977) and Lacan and as the mystics of a variety of religious traditions propose, our search for answers should always acknowledge the ineffable within it (Webb & Sells, 1995).

The tension then between our faith of pursuing our incompletion and the anxiety that this incompletion causes leaves all of us susceptible to slipping back to positions that feel safer but less open. In times of social tumult, there is tremendous anxiety about the available resources for the ongoing-ness of our being and that of our loved ones. Indeed, there might not even need to be cataclysmic events like war when national leaders callously exploit our anxiety of being incomplete by simply proclaiming that we are existentially threatened. Defining some "other" as a threat to our "way of life" is often enough to rally those of us whose embrace of the otherness is tenuous into feeling that a threat to our being-ness is at hand. We are prodded to feel that if our worldview does not prevail, and by "prevail" is often meant "dominate," then we will not survive. When this happens, the perspectives of others become heretical and dangerous. In other words, context is lost and ignored, and those who were appreciated as "others" by us now once again become simply, flat "not-me's."

In this devolution, we become good, and they become bad, and, as Orwell points out, "[C]ompetitive prestige" (1945/2018, p. 4) becomes the rule of the day, because with prestige comes privilege and power to prevail. When this happens,

> [A]ctions are held to be good or bad, not on their own merits, but according to who does them, and there is almost no kind of outrage – torture, the use of hostages, forced labour, mass deportations, imprisonment without trial, forgery, assassination, the bombing of civilians – which does not change its moral color when it is committed by 'our' side. (1945/2018, p. 13)

Patriotism and the depressive position

Orwell's patriotism is the less viral version of tribalism, and within the foundation we have established regarding existential-relational positions, we propose that it reflects movement toward the depressive position, though not necessarily the attainment of it. Recall that within this position there is appreciation of the otherness of others, even if it does not entail yet the transcendent appreciation of one-ness within otherness (difference). In the movement from nationalism to patriotism, there is an implicit appreciation that the patriot that I am is different than the patriot that you are. Orwell makes clear that we, as the patriot, are committed to our "faith" and want our community to reflect this worldview. However, we also recognize that others have different faiths with ramifications for how their communities function. There is a nascent mentality of live and let live, a kind of "I am me" and "you are you."

Imagining a third option: Internationalism

The tribalism that goes beyond patriotism is a tribalism where we can imagine a kind of internationalist perspective, a perspective where, simplistically stated, we hold the tension between different-ness and same-ness, a perspective where we embrace how we are both different from and the same as others. This kind of tribalism reflects an existential position that in some fundamental ways seeks to upend the typical understanding of tribes as boundaried groups.

What happens when patriotism and nationalism collide?

The rub in our discussion of tribes, of course, comes when for one reason or another one community feels its existence to be threatened. That "letting them live" will mean that "we won't live." When this fundamental anxiety takes hold, the reigning mentality of a society is that we must rule or perish (Friedman, 2011, unnumbered), and the draw of the paranoid-schizoid position again becomes a factor. In our "faith" and our "fear," we descend into the binary of good and bad, a place where our goodness is as obvious to us as is the badness of those who aren't us, the "not-me's." With the sense that our existence is at stake, we seek to destroy before being destroyed. Orwell says of the nationalist that in his effort to prevail it is "impossible [for him or her] ... to conceal his [sic] allegiance. The smallest slur upon his own unit, or any implied praise of a rival organization, fills him with uneasiness which he can only relieve by making some sharp retort" (1945/2018, p. 9). In short, there is a descent into tooth and claw mentality.

Crucially, it takes only one tribe to feel it is in existential jeopardy for the tooth and claw mentality to be a factor of importance. Of course, if two tribes convergently feel this jeopardy, tribal warfare blossoms. This warfare can manifest as actual war or as some metaphorical dramatization of it. Furthermore, in this tribal warfare, it is not necessarily the case that both tribes will be in a paranoid-schizoid position, a position in which it feels to a tribe that its truth is the truth. It *can*, however, be the case that both tribes are in this position, and if so, the tooth and claw battle will be certain to be a snarl of intense, even deadly proportions.

However, if both are not in the paranoid-schizoid position, the tribe that is in the depressive position is faced with a truly difficult decision about how to respond to the destructive intent of the paranoid-schizoid tribe. Recall that Orwell describes the patriot (the aspiring depressive position) tribe as by "its nature defensive, both militarily and culturally" (1945/2018, p. 2). The question will be how to defend.

One obvious defense, already noted earlier, is the paranoid-schizoid one where we enter into the tooth and claw. We abandon our usual existential-relational position and jump into the trench with the paranoid-schizoid tribe. But there can also, at least logically, be defenses that reflect a depressive or transcendent position. It is a perspective that is more lightly captured in a phrase than befits the seriousness of our subject and yet a phrase which speaks aptly to the point: we must decide "when to hold them and when to fold them." We hasten to say that this phrase is not offered as a disguised plea for pacifism. Pacifism, too, as Orwell notes, can be tribal. Pacifists are as susceptible as any other group to tribalistic thinking and to the arrogance that comes when we forgot that we are tribes of faith. That said, a pacifist stance is, of course, one that the depressive position tribe might adopt.

Other stances we can hold

Other stances we might hold entail our ability to achieve and sustain a hold on the transcendental existential position. In this position, we recognize the complexity of our being-ness. We recognize that we all have multiple facets to our identities, whether we realize it or not. In other words, we all have the potential for affiliation with a number of tribes. We need not be subsumed by any particular one if we can embrace the transcendent awareness that none of us is only one thing. As such, we have choice about how to respond to an attack by a paranoid-schizoid tribe.

The attack that comes to our doorstep from the paranoid-schizoid tribe entails an assertion that we are of another tribe, a tribe that is named in some unworthy way and done so to underline that we are *not-them* (not of their tribe). In other words, an important part of the attack is one of definition. The nationalist tribe in needing to assert itself labels and defines the other in such a way as to remove their complexities and multitude of belonging; the other is in some particular way unsavory and thus dangerous. We are the outsider, and the outsider is dangerous.

Once we've started in the war of naming, we are perhaps bound to be stuck in a doer-done-to (Benjamin, 2004) paranoid-schizoid enactment. It is easy to lose focus and remain stuck with asserting who we are. Through doing this, we play our role in a feedback cycle. Even as we serve to differentiate ourselves from those who seek to name us, we affirm to those others the very ways we are different from them. They do not see this difference as positive but rather as an affirmation of our threat. So gripped are they in trying to define, they lose the ability to hear and listen.

There is, however, an alternative reaction to meeting the paranoid-schizoid attack with attack in kind. In this reaction, we forbear from granting any authority to paranoid-schizoid tribe to define our essence or to name us. This is not asserted through a counter-accusation or through descent into some wormhole of debate about names. Instead, it is asserted in an *action* which, with or without words, says, "I am more than that." It is, in other words, an action that embodies one of the basic postulates of humanistic psychology (Greening, 2006) that we, as human beings, supersede the sum of our parts and cannot be reduced to components. In the developmental parlance of this chapter, it is a position that reflects a positioning within a depressive or transcendent position that demonstrates an appreciation of the multiplicity of our being-ness. This allows us relative insulation against a bombardment of some specific and simplistic categorization or naming.

We can adopt this depressive or transcendent positioning *if,* in the face of the paranoid-schizoid arrogant (anxious) presumption of knowing truth, we do not become reactively arrogant. If we *do* so, especially in a knee-jerk way, we have failed to consider context, and, consequently, we will forget that we can decide whether to "hold or fold." In other words, we can only decide if there is something we can do only *if* we recognize that we have the authority to name the rules of the game on our own terms. Thus, we might choose to enter into more of what might seem like a paranoid-schizoid position, forcefully but tentatively as a reflection our ability to name ourselves in response to what feels threatening. In the position, we may need to adapt some of its mentality in order to move ahead and respond to the aggression at our doorstep. However, as we do so as a matter of choice of our own naming, we preserve an important aspect of the depressive position and so hold the potential for also exiting the paranoid-schizoid position. Accordingly, as stated, achieving this is a complicated business, we note the possibility to hold and exercise *our* authority in defining ourselves.

To illustrate this point, we recall Luigi Pirandello's *The Rules of the Game* (1962). In this play, Leone underlines the ultimate relativity of the social rules to which we subscribe, often with little conscious awareness. In the story Leone agrees to the terms for fighting a sword duel, terms which include a provision that his "second" must fight for him if he reneges. So embedded is the expectation that honor will prevail with an agreement to duel that no one even considers the possibility that Leone will not fight. To not fight would be to accept more dishonor than is bearable. Of course, Leone refuses; he "folds." Guido, whom Leone has named as his "second" and who is also his romantic rival, cannot muster a corresponding appreciation of the relativity of naming that ensues in our tribal allegiances. He fights the duel and dies.

The draw of the paranoid-schizoid position is very strong,

especially when we feel threatened by otherness. As Audre Lorde (1984) reasonably says,

> We have all been programmed to respond to the human differences between us with fear and loathing and to handle that difference in one of three ways: ignore it, and if that is not possible, copy it if we think it dominant, or destroy it if we think it is subordinate. (p. 115)

In this regard, we highlight the possibility of deconstructing and re-constructing who we are, of developing new iterations of how we occupy space in the world. Within the postulates of humanistic psychology, we might say that we affirm our intentionality as beings, beings who can cause things to happen and beings who "seek meaning, value, and creativity" (Greening, 2006, p. 239).

Examples of the collision between nationalism and patriotism

We again turn to Kendi (2019) to help us consider how this collision between nationalism and patriotism has been playing out within our current social context. In his exposition on racism, Kendi grapples with what is helpful in confronting other's and one's own racism. He essentially says that rather than simply descend into shame, a view we think is akin to surrendering to anxiety about one's own badness (Chapter 4) we must consider that in our racism we are always both a victim and victimizer. Utilizing metaphor (Brown, 2020) to fasten his point, he says that we grow up from our earliest days victimized by the "rain" of racist policies and constructions of meaning that fall upon and wet us to our core. We then victimize others with the results of this rain.

Clearly speaking from a transcendent position, Kendi says that the good news is that "No one is essentially racist" (Brown, 2020, 48:00). That in other words, no one's being is entirely racist. Realizing this, confessing our victimizing and looking for an umbrella to protect ourselves we can work to be antiracist. In short, we can realize that there are rules of the game that are always in play and always being written. Thus, while these rules may stem from societal structures, it is within our capacities as reflective human beings to recognize how these rules shape our actions so that we can choose to find ways of not adhering to them and instead adhere to a different set of rules. Although "the powerful play goes on ... [we] may contribute a verse" (Whitman, 1926, p. 229). We have available to us both choice and the responsibility inherent to it (Greening, 2006, p. 239).

Looting in Minneapolis and Black Lives Matter

Moving from the abstract to the more particular we can get closer to the world that Kendi is addressing so forthrightly by focusing on the tumultuous real world at our feet. Recent examples of events in the United States help us illustrate the results that ensue when paranoid-schizoid tribalism (a) isn't recognized as prevailing or (b) is the prevailing interpretative perspective in the face of a plea for recognition of otherness. For the former, we will look at the looting that occurred in Minneapolis. For the latter, we will consider some of what prevents people from saying "Black lives matter."

Looting occurred during the Minneapolis protests over the death of George Floyd, a death caused by the nearly 9-minute pinning of policeman Derek Chauvin's knee against his neck. In reference to this, Trevor Noah, in one of his recent "social distancing shows" (2020), makes a provocative and poignant comment about this. He essentially says that when the community's implicit social contract is broken, the pertinent perspective is not how looting *doesn't* make sense but how it *does* make sense.

Noah goes on to say that time and again black people witness that those in power kill them and do not abide by the contract to protect them. Implicitly, we think that Noah is pointing here to the paranoid-schizoid tribalism that allows some police to view black deaths as less significant, less significant, because their otherness has been flattened and defined, consciously or unconsciously, as those who are "not us" and thus here to disrupt our tribe, our welfare. Hence, atrocities can occur with the expectation that nothing much in the way of consequences will ensue. For example, a recent article that summarizes the findings of the *National Violent Death Reporting System, 17 U.S. States, 2009-2012* (DeGue et al., 2016) highlights the structural inequities that demonstrate these paranoid-schizoid stances. Specifically, that

Victims were majority [W]hite (52%) but disproportionately [B] lack (32%) with a fatality rate 2.8 times higher among [B]lacks than [W]hites. Most victims were reported to be armed (83%); however [B]lack victims were more likely to be unarmed (14.8%) than [W]hite (9.8%) or Hispanic (5.8%) victims. (p. 173)

Noah's provocative take on the sense we can make of looting essentially calls attention to the fact that the systematic racism that the findings suggest stems from a paranoid-schizoid position that does not support a true commitment to recognizing that "Black lives matter." From Noah's perspective, then, it stands to reason that at least some Blacks will also adopt a paranoid-schizoid position. That they will feel themselves to be in the tooth and claw crisis and so will attack the livelihood of those who stand in the established order of society that allows these "rules of the game." We think it interesting to consider here that when people argue about rightness and wrongness of actions and do so by convergence to a paranoid-schizoid position, they engage essentially in a moral equivalency debate, a debate which speaks past any concern for the ideal of right and wrong with some version of: "Since you did *that*, I am justified in doing *this.*" This is a transactional mode of operation that is often associated with Donald Trump and that we will see demonstrated in our next example.

Our second example continues with the theme of "Black lives matter," and how leaders can exploit our existential vulnerabilities. We quote the words of former Vice President Mike Pence and former President Donald Trump. When Pence is asked several times by a news correspondent about whether he can say that Black lives matter, Pence delimits himself to "All lives matter in a very real sense" (Taff, 2020, June 20, 1:41–1:42). Pence goes on to say, "Well, I don't accept the fact … that there's a segment of American society that disagrees in the preciousness and importance of every human life" (Taff, 2020, June 20, 3:25–3:36). Some days later when Trump is asked by another correspondent why so many Blacks in the United States are being killed during engagements with police officers, Trump, embodying the moral transactional and equivalency position that we note above, answers, "So are White people. So are White people. What a terrible question to ask. So are White people. More White people, by the way, more White people" (Herridge, 2020, July 14, 3:08–3:22).

In Pence's and Trump's words, we hear the paranoid-schizoid position in full steam and the appeal to their followers to organize around tribal ideas. Orwell pegs it, especially Trump's reaction. Speaking of the nationalist, Orwell says, "The smallest slur ... or any implied praise of a rival organization, fills him [the nationalist] with uneasiness which he can only relieve by making some sharp retort" (1945/2018, p. 9). From the binary that the paranoid-schizoid position exemplifies, there is no capability to hold to a perspective which overarches one's own interests (needs) and those of another (others). Hence, neither Pence nor Trump can or will hold in their consideration the otherness of black lives, which makes the context of the movement powerful and significant (see Hoffman et al., 2016, for an examination of the history of the movement).

Instead, they fixate, respectively, on "every human life" and "White people" as if there is an impossible conjunction between Black lives mattering and other (their own) lives mattering. In doing this, they effectively locate themselves as within the paranoid-schizoid position, and, more insidiously, they attempt to rally their followers to adapt this position as well. Pence goes so far as to implicitly characterize Black Lives Matter supporters as people who do not value the "preciousness and importance of every human life" (3:34–3:36). In this move, there is a denial of the otherness of the other in a broad claim that in essence attempts to invalidate their message. In so doing, Black Lives Matter is treated as a threatening outside group to be erased and not held. It is here that we see the dangerous overlay of psychology and politics, as the move toward nationalism ("human lives" and "White lives") is clearly political but operates at a psychological level.

Trump and Pence implicitly understand that the simplistic paranoid-schizoid good-bad view of the world has power. Consciously or not, they grasp that tribes seek loyal subscription of their membership and seek a sense of a "tribal us" to override disciplined appreciation of the worthy otherness of those in other tribes. Indeed, holding onto the otherness of others gets in the way of the paranoid-schizoid purpose of classification, since it does not translate easily in a way which seems forthrightly to serve this bonding purpose. That said that which is our *tendency* need not be seen as our *destiny*. We have the opportunity to make choices about how we view and respond to others. Speaking of "nationalistic loves and hatreds," Orwell says,

> [T]hey are a part of the make-up of most of us. Whether it is possible to get rid of them I do no know, but ... it is possible to struggle against them, and that this is essentially a *moral* effort. (1945/2018, original italics, p. 30)

We can do this when we anchor ourselves in a depressive or transcendent existential-relational position, a position wherein our appreciation of other-ness and context go hand in hand. We can thus choose to realize that Black lives matter and "all lives matter" are not oppositional and that emphasizing one is not at the expense of the other. Indeed, while not the point, we think our ability to say Black Lives Matter more powerfully lifts up all lives as it recognizes the interrelatedness of self and other.

In our college and university communities

While in this chapter we have focused *beyond* the contexts our university and college communities, we think that our assertions about the connections between tribalism and existential-relational positions clearly pertains to issues *within* our communities. As we have noted especially in Chapters 6 and 7, institutions, consciously or otherwise, sometimes offer themselves as the path for how students can seek important *completion* as emerging adults. In doing this, we as "ongoing" members of our institutional community can struggle deeply when we feel that we disappoint or fail our students who are the new members of our community. While, as stated frequently, this failing is sometimes a crucial part of our developmental processes, nonetheless, this sense of disappointing or failing can be a challenge for us to find peace with.

This can be especially true when we think about our cultural identifications and the structures to which we are all subject. Then we have to hold the tension between the ways that these structures and our participation within them delimit our views in ways which are racist, ableist, sexist or, otherwise, narrowed by some kind of "ist" or "ism." In other words, that embedded "ism's" rain down upon us is something which we always must have the courage to acknowledge if we want to maintain our integrity and be able to be the educating and agentic community of change that we see seek to be. In fact, our coming to peace with this is something that we, as authors, think is an essential aspect of the learning that we want to provide and exemplify to our students. (There is, of course, important parallels of this challenge with what as parents we face in raising a child who is inevitably different from us with their needs and views of who they and we are.)

At the same time, part of coming to peace is the other side of this tension. Beyond acknowledging our various "isms," we as institutional members for various reasons may all be subject to conditions where we struggle to tolerate and embrace difference. This includes the ways that we try to embrace our various "isms" and how we work to create change in our societies (local and global). So, when for whatever reason we cannot tolerate difference or challenge, there is, as Orwell reminds us, a danger of devolving into the "nationalistic/paranoid-schizoid" position where "intellectual decencies can vanish, the past can be altered, and the plainest fact can be denied" (1945/2018, p. 27).

So, while we as institutions may proclaim views that indicate we wholeheartedly support diversity and otherness, our realization of these views in our policies and practices can be myopic. Moreover, while we may not see them as myopic, they may be differently experienced by other community members and especially our students. If we as members of the institutional community can acknowledge this and with depressive position spirit accept that our humanity dictates that we disappoint others and fall short in always being aligned with what is "good and right," then we can better hope that we can hold with mindful appreciation the otherness of community members who take issue with how the community has embodied (institutionalized) itself.

Conversely, if we falter into paranoid position anxiety about being "bad" and destructive, then we are at risk of making the "unforced errors" that accompany our defensive needs as an institution to deny or compensate for our being caught in the structural rain of an "ism."

We are at risk of being unable to adjust our heartily embraced institutional self-perception so that we can point ourselves toward a truer "north," which can only be achieved through fully embracing our shortcomings and not quickly attempting to mollify and appease.

This speaks to a final challenge, where in our efforts to align ourselves more truly toward our ideal institutional characterization, we can easily get caught between a depressive and paranoid-schizoid position where we are susceptible to thinking that *goodness* that disappoints is *badness*. When this happens, staying in open, meaning-making conversation with others, especially with students who voice the challenge to our self-perception, is enormously trying. In these times we as an institution easily can devolve into a "nationalism" that implicitly or explicitly arrogantly asserts that we are the older, wiser, more educated tribe within the community with historical bona fides. Similarly, in feeling our "badness," we may react from a "guilt reaction" regarding our own human shortcomings. This can lead to knee-jerk reactions to return to the good, including mollifications and false promises. These come too easily and do not address the hurt but rather paste over it.

If, by contrast, we can reach toward being more "global" in our perspective, we can adhere to recognition that disappointment and loss are a part of the naming and renaming that marks the incompletion which we all face, whether as an institutional or as individual. From here, we can return to the perspective and need for radical dialogue with not just students but also others who hold different views. With such adherence, we can emerge out of being politically "stuck" and more rightfully claim to be "activists."

Summary and concluding thoughts

Black Lives Matter is a political movement; so, it is susceptible to tribalism in all its possibilities just as any movement is. As such there are undoubtedly members that function from a paranoid-schizoid position and others who do not. However, we, all of us in society and regardless of our color (but especially we who are not black), have the challenge of what choice we make in how we cast the functioning of this tribe. If we see the tribe as a group consumed by paranoid-schizoid positioning, we will be inclined to hear in the slogan, "Black lives matter" that "Only black lives matter." Especially as Whites in America, Kendi asserts that we can easily fall into this perspective because we can take some actions of members within the Black Lives Matter movement as emblematic of all members of it. As Kendi says of white racism, "We generalize the individual negativities of persons of color while we individualize the individual negativities of White people" (Brown, 2020, minute 17).

If we fall into this paranoid-schizoid/nationalistic tribalism, we begin to dance with a tooth and claw reaction. We will do as Mike Pence and Donald Trump felt compelled to do. We will hear the assertion that black lives matter as "my life doesn't matter because I'm not Black," and we will *not* be able to nod in emphatic sympathy and say in heartfelt agreement that "Yes, Black lives matter." Instead, we will feel compelled to say some insistent version of "All lives matter," as if this truth were not obvious or as if this truth were in jeopardy. Accordingly, we can recognize how wet have are from being in the rain without an umbrella, and we have a chance to fortify ourselves in a transcendent position where we recognize that our tribe is everyone's tribe, that we are all in this together.

By way of concluding example, we are reminded of a brief story from our particular institution's history. Former president, Jack Coleman, learned that angry students planned to demonstrate their outrage at US policy that sustained a war in Vietnam by burning the American flag. Coleman joined the students in their rally on the front green, engaged them in conversation about their impassioned views and then invited them to wash the flag instead of burning it. Coleman and the students found a way to make meaning together. In washing rather than burning, they moved beyond the paranoid binary. Washing the flag was their symbolic way of acknowledging that the war policy and its misguided nature was dirtying the principles and integrity not only of "bad guys" in Washington but also of all of us over whom the flag was flying.

Note

1 This chapter is a version of a previous publication: Webb, R.E. & Rosenbaum, P.J. (2021). Tribalism: Where George Orwell leads us and where an understanding of existential-relational positions extends us. Published online on 5 March. *Theory & Psychology.* http://doi.org/10.1177/0959354321998776

References

Benjamin, J (2004). Beyond does and done to: An intersubjective view of third ness. *The Psychoanalytic Quarterly*, *73* (1), 5–46. 10.1002/j.2167-4 086.2004.tb0015.x

Bion, W (1977). *Seven servants: Four works by Wilfred R. Bion.* Jason Aronson.

Brown, B (Host). (2020, June 3). Brené with Ibram X. Kendi on how to be an antiracist [Audio podcast episode]. In *Unlocking us with Brené Brown.* https://brenebrown.com/podcast/brene-with-ibram-x-kendi-on-how-to-be-an-antiracist/. (Brené Brown, PhD, MSW is a research professor at the University of Houston).

Clark, C, Liu, B, Winegard, B, & Ditto, P (2019). Tribalism is human nature. *Current Directions in Psychological Science*, *28*(6), 587–592. 10.11 77/0963721419862289.

Clark, CJ , & Winegard, BM (2020). Tribalism in war and peace: The nature and evolution of ideological epistemology and its significance for modern social science. *Psychological Inquiry*, *31*(1), 1–22. https://doi.org/1 0.1080/1047840X.2020.1721233

DeGue, S, Fowler, KA, & Calkins, C (2016). Deaths due to use of lethal force by law enforcement, Findings from the National Violent Death Reporting System, 17 U.S. States, 20009-2012. *Journal of Preventive Medicine*, *51* (5), 173–187. https://doi.org/

Ditto, PH, Liu, B, Clark, CJ, Wojcik, SP, Chen, EE, Grady, RH, Celniker, J & Zinger, JF (2018). At least bias is bipartisan: A meta-analytic comparison of partisan bias in liberals and conservatives. *Perspectives on Psychological Science*, *14* (2), 273–291. 10.1177/1745691617746796.

Felman, S (1987). *Jacques Lacan and the adventure of insight.* Harvard University Press.

Friedman, T (2011, April 19). Future in the Middle East is a case of pray, hope, prepare. *East Bay Times.* https://www.eastbaytimes.com/2011/04/19/thomas-friedman-future-in-the-middle-east-is-a-case-of-pray-hope-prepare/.

Gellner, E (2006). *Nations and Nationalism, 2nd edition.* Cornell University Press. (Original work published 1983)

Gonzalez, F (2016). On the relation to non-relationality. *Psychoanalytic Dialogues*, *26* (5), 522–531. 10.1080/10481889909539308

Gordon, A (1967). Six hours with Rudyard Kipling. *The Kipling Journal, V. XXXIV*, *162* (June), 5–8. https://www.kiplingjournal.com/textfiles/KJ162. text (Original work published 1935).

Greening, T (2006). Five basic postulates of humanistic psychology. *Journal of Humanistic Psychology*, *46* (3), 239. 10.1177/002216780604600301.

Kendi, IX (2019). *How to be an antiracist*. One World.

Herridge, C (2020, July 15). Transcript: Trump on masks, reopening schools, race and pardoning Roger Stone. *CBS News*. https://www. cbsnews/news/trump-race-face-mask-school-roger-stone/.

Hesse, H (1929). *Steppenwolf*. (B Creighton, Trans.) Henry Holt and Company.

Hoffman, L Granger, N, Vallejos, L, & Moats, M (2016). An existential-humanistic perspective on Black Lives Matter and contemporary protests movements. *Journal of Humanistic Psychology*, *56* (6), 595–611. 10.1177/ 0022167816652273.

Lacan, J (1968). *Speech and language in psychoanalysis* (A Wilden, Trans.). Johns Hopkins University Press. (Original work published 1956).

Lorde, A (1984). *Sister outsider: Essays and speeches*. Crossing Press.

Lacan, J (1978). *The four fundamental concepts of psychoanalysis* (J Miller, Ed. & A Sheridan, Trans.). Norton. (Original work published 1956).

Noah, T [The Daily Show with Trevor Noah]. (2020, May 29). *George Floyd, Minneapolis, Ahmaud Arbery & Amy Cooper* [Video]. YouTube. https://www.youtube.com/watch?v=v4amCf-VbA_c.

Orwell, G (2010). *Homage to Catalonia*. Houghton Mifflin Harcourt. (Original work published 1938).

Orwell, G (2018). *Notes on nationalism*. Penguin Books. (Originally published 1945).

Pirandello, L (1962). *To clothe the naked and two other plays* (W Murray, Trans., pp. 77–140). Dutton.

Sartre, J-P (1966). *Being and nothingness, a phenomenological essay on ontology* (HE Barnes, Trans.) Washington Square Press. (Original work published 1943).

Storr, A (1996). *Feet of clay, saints, sinners, and madmen: A study of gurus*. Free Press.

Taff, B (June 20, 2020). 6ABC news Brian Taff interviews Vice President Mike Pence on Black Lives Matter movement, coronavirus. *6abc*. https://6abc. com/mike-pence-black-lives-matter-all-interview-juneteenth/6256371/.

Tong, K & von Hippel, W (2020). Sexual selection, history, and the evolution of tribalism. *Psychological Inquiry*, *31* (1), 23–25 10.1080/104784 0X.2020.1722580.

Webb, RE & Sells, MA (1995). Lacan and Bion, Psychoanalysis and the mystical language of 'unsaying'. *Theory & Psychology*, *5* (2), 195–215. 10.1177/0959354395052002.

Whitman, W (1926). *Leaves of Grass: O me! O life!* Doubleday & Company. (Original work published 1892).

Concluding Thoughts: What about the Rest of Adolescence?

The importance of psychological process

Throughout this volume we have attempted to demonstrate how thinking about adolescents' situatedness from an existential-relational perspective can help us to make sense of their conduct in their world and to engage meaningfully with them in therapy. Our model, which has emerged over our years of collaborative discussion and writings, emphasizes processes and periods of development. The four developmental positions we describe draw from a blend of object relations, interpersonal psychoanalysis, cultural psychology and existential philosophy. These positions establish our foundation for the ways we come relate to self and other as we become agentic beings in the world with unique identities, desires and values. They are structured and mediated through culture, both our immediate familial and the broader and more societal. Semiotics or signs provide a basis for agentic and active meaning making and engagement in the world. They provide the basis for our co-constructive understanding of self and other. These are bidirectional relationships. We are both shaped by and shaping culture (Valsiner, 2009).

Accordingly, these processes are also susceptible to all forms of interference, stagnation, dysregulation, hyper-generalization and so forth. We as beings are limitless in our capacity to construct novel meanings that orient us toward creative growth *and* stagnating delimitation, both of which play importantly in how we relate both to others and ourselves. In this, we have offered numerous theoretical and case examples of some of what we think causes problems in our

DOI: 10.4324/9781003246558-10

ongoing processes of becoming. We hope to have adequately shown that far from being the result of "bad actors" or "parents" that these semiotic processes are complex, causing all of us to grapple with existential anxieties related to who we are. Moreover, they are subject to structural and societal factors, including, but not limited to class, race, gender, sexuality, neuro-cognitive functioning, and histories of trauma that set very real parameters and boundaries.

While we have focused upon how these structural and inter-personal issues can be expressed within our relationships, especially during our early years, our intent, as we noted earlier, has been to articulate where we think problems arise in our developmental process. This helps us to have a sense of how to develop and sustain relationships when these individuals become our patients. More broadly, it also helps inform the perspective we hold as community members at institutions where we are always planning for how to meet the educational needs of the "whole" student.

In thinking about the ways we emerge and become active subjects, we are able to create and sustain relationships with people of different backgrounds, identities and social locations. While we must be sensitive to difference, we can also go beyond this toward curiosity and a full-throated embrace of it. This is something that proceeds naturally because recognizing the boundaries between ourselves and others fundamentally entails discernment of the similarity between ourselves and others. We maintain that our processual approach to in-completeness, incongruity, fluidity of being, the unconscious and uncertainty in the ever-going journey of becoming helps in our work with a wide range of adolescents. Adolescence and emerging adult-hood is, of course, the pot in which acute and open sensitivity to similarity and difference seems so reliably to stir.

We think our approach differs from other contemporary view-points of adolescence, identity development, multicultural competence, psychotherapy and so forth. We are concerned that other viewpoints too easily devolve into static, positivistic, cognitive and modular models that attempt to classify and organize aspects of being into variables to be tested, measured and assessed. While this type of "knowing" does have value, we find that it significantly constrains the way we consider the complexities and challenges of *becoming* both in adolescence and beyond.

Indeed, we argue that the complexities of adolescence and emerging adulthood, however uniquely flavored, are also a part of the broader journey of life that we all must embrace. In this, we may be seen as thinking of adolescents as "young adults," which to a certain extent is true. They are precisely "young" not necessarily by way of age (though this too) but more in their relative "newness" to the process of becoming. This newness affords them a valued and unique perspective which we think more conventional models of adolescence tend to reify into static conceptions that do not befit the dynamic vitality that characterizes this period in our development. We hope the developmental perspective that we offer challenges us to think about and feel the complex wonderfulness of adolescence so that we can work more relationally with our students. We are convinced that engaging them successfully clinically and, in all contexts, does not grow out of viewing them as "big children" or "small adults" but rather as "younger versions of ourselves."

Finding our way to adolescents

Our view of psychological development as an open-ended process is crucial to how we relate to adolescents and emerging adults. With this view, we understand that we have as much to learn from them as they do from us, and that what most matters is that we find our way to them as fellow travelers in the world, fellow beings. This is especially crucial within the context of institutes of higher education. While adolescents are the very lifeblood that sustains our post-secondary institutions and eventually make up our ever-important alumni, they are also rather temporary residents. In other words, though they live and breathe the same university air that we do as counselors, deans and administrators, they are also very much on "our turf" when they meet with us. Our duration (Bergson, 1907/1944) as part of the institute ensures this. Thus, it is incumbent upon us to "reach" for them if that is what is necessary in order to "find them."

This process and approach of finding our way toward our adolescent patients reminds us of D.W. Winnicott's description of hide and seek (1975). Specifically, he writes "it is a joy to be hidden and a disaster not to be found" (p. 187). In other words, we need insulating privacy so that we can explore life and grow at our own pace, but, as social beings, we also yearn to be discovered. Our important care-givers and loved ones have to not only seek us out and find us but we also cannot be so well-hidden, so guarded and defended, that we do not allow ourselves to be found.

Áporos of this, a queer, straight, Caucasian male, dealing with tremendous anxiety about graduating college described a story of playing hide and seek during his early elementary school years. He had hidden himself up in a tree so well that no one had a chance of finding him. He stayed up there through the calls to go inside, hoping to be found by someone. Somehow, the teachers failed to account for him and so from his perch he observed everyone go inside. He waited for as long as he could – an indeterminate period in his recollection. When he finally went down and went inside, he learned that he had missed a birthday celebration, which included cake. He was crest-fallen to have not been found and to miss out on the celebration.

What it means to look, what it means to hide, what it means to search, find and be found all shift in the different ways we move throughout our lifespan. In this, we anticipate our own evolution and change of how we go about relating and thinking about adolescents. It is from this perspective that we hope to have engaged you as a reader and also to have demonstrated theory that is sensitive to process, becoming, identity and change. That this may also mirror how we relate to others as a parent, friend or colleague makes this all the more relevant.

Unanswered questions, unexplored topics

We recognize that in the application of our process to different aspects of adolescence some readers may be left wondering about other aspects that we have not covered. What about sex, hookups, relationships, friendships, drugs and alcohol, sports, video games, clubs, academics, procrastination, perfectionism, imposter syndrome, resource scarcity, the job market, religion and so forth? In this book, we most certainly have not addressed many things relevant to adolescence. In some ways, limitations in space have disallowed us this opportunity. Hence, to the interested reader, we direct you to some of our other publications (Webb & Rosenbaum, 2019; 2018; Webb & Birky, 2021; Rosenbaum, 2013; 2010). However, we hasten to say that our falling short of being as comprehensive in our approach as others might wish also simply reflects the fact that we are "still thinking on the matter." With this book as with life we cannot be all things; our becoming some-things means that other things are foreclosed, at least temporarily as naming, un-naming and re-naming proceeds. In our case, "re-naming" might be our gathering ourselves together for another volume. Time will tell.

In any case, the topics that we have chosen to bring to the forefront in this book are the ones that feel most urgent to us at this point in time. Our written offering about destructive processes, suicide, trauma, otherness and groups all feel crucial to us within the current zeitgeist. While certainly, love, sex and money are also important, they do not feel like the topics that clinicians struggle with so urgently. Moreover, they usually are not the issues that cause the community anxieties that clearly arise when the concern is about suicide, trauma, diversity or group affiliations.

Hence, we felt it worthwhile to focus ourselves in this book on what we have found most challenging to ourselves and our colleagues in our work and community membership on campus. More times than we can enumerate the issues that we discuss in this book have been the substance, subtextually or manifestly, of our personal morning chats, phone calls and consultations with each other. In our grappling to understand and ground ourselves, we have relished the journey we have taken both into the nitty-gritty of everyday functioning *and* the soaring heights of theory and philosophy. We look forward to the further evolution of that grappling, and we hope it will involve dialogue with our readers.

References

Bergson, H (1907/1944). *Creative evolution*. Random House Modern Library.

Rosenbaum, PJ (2013). The role of projective identification in constructing the "Other": Why do Westerners want to "liberate" Muslim women? *Culture & Psychology, 19* (2), 213–224. 10.1177/1354067×12456719

Rosenbaum, PJ (2010). Deception in adolescent sexual conduct. *Integrative Psychological and Behavioral Sciences, 44* (4), 370–380. 10.1007/s12124-010-9141-8

Valsiner, J (2009). Cultural psychology today: Innovations and oversights. *Culture & Psychology, 15* (1), 5–39. 10.1177/1354067x08101427

Webb, RE & Birky, I (2021). Meditation on the Occasion of Tragic Loss: Friendship and Incompleteness, *Journal of College Student Psychotherapy*, DOI: 10.1080/87568225.2021.1890297

Webb, RE & Rosenbaum, PJ (2019) Resilience and thinking Perpendicularly: A meditation or morning jog. *Journal of College Student Psychotherapy, 33* (1), 75–88, DOI: 10.1080/87568225.2018.1449687

Webb, R & Rosenbaum, PJ (2018). The variety of procrastination: With different existential positions different reasons for it. *Integrative Psychological and Behavioral Sciences*. Advance online publication. 10.1 007/s12124-018-9467-1

Winnicott, DW (1971). *Playing and reality*. Routledge Press.

Index